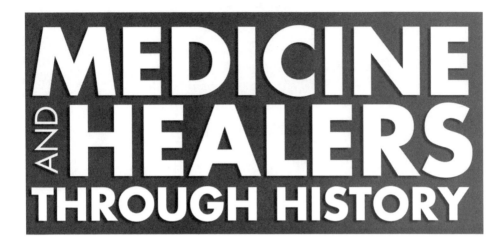

MEDICINE AND HEALERS THROUGH HISTORY

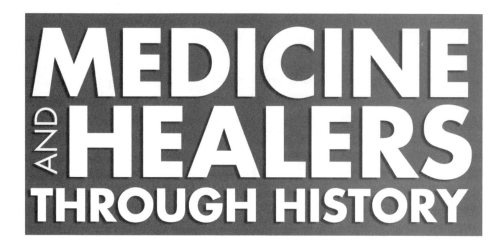

MEDICINE AND HEALERS THROUGH HISTORY

EDITED BY KARA ROGERS, SENIOR EDITOR, BIOMEDICAL SCIENCES

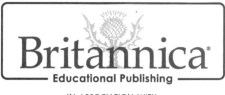

Britannica®
Educational Publishing

IN ASSOCIATION WITH

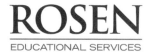

ROSEN
EDUCATIONAL SERVICES

Published in 2011 by Britannica Educational Publishing
(a trademark of Encyclopædia Britannica, Inc.)
in association with Rosen Educational Services, LLC
29 East 21st Street, New York, NY 10010.

First Edition

Britannica Educational Publishing
Michael I. Levy: Executive Editor
J.E. Luebering: Senior Manager
Marilyn L. Barton: Senior Coordinator, Production Control
Steven Bosco: Director, Editorial Technologies
Lisa S. Braucher: Senior Producer and Data Editor
Yvette Charboneau: Senior Copy Editor
Kathy Nakamura: Manager, Media Acquisition
Kara Rogers: Senior Editor, Biomedical Sciences

Rosen Educational Services
Alexandra Hanson-Harding: Editor
Nelson Sá: Art Director
Cindy Reiman: Photography Manager
Nicole Russo: Designer
Matthew Cauli: Cover Design
Introduction by Catherine Vanderhoof

Library of Congress Cataloging-in-Publication Data

Medicine and healers through history / edited by Kara Rogers.—1st ed.
    p. ; cm.—(Health and disease in society)
"In association with Britannica Educational Publishing, Rosen Educational Services."
Includes bibliographical references and index.
ISBN 978-1-61530-367-0 (library binding)
1. Physicians—Biography. 2. Medicine—History. I. Rogers, Kara. II. Series: Health and
disease in society.
  [DNLM: 1. History of Medicine—Encyclopedias—English. 2. Disease—history—
Encyclopedias—English. 3. Health Personnel—history--Encyclopedias—English. WZ 13]
R134.M37 2011
610.9—dc22

                                                              2010029135

Manufactured in the United States of America

Cover Shutterstock.com

On pages 1, 26, 55, 76, 96, 116, 135, 160, 185: This X-ray image of a chest shows a growth
on the left side, which might indicate lung cancer. *National Cancer Institute*

CONTENTS

6

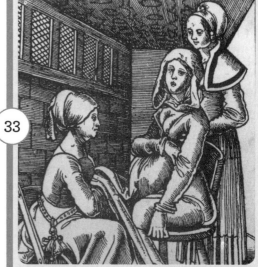

33

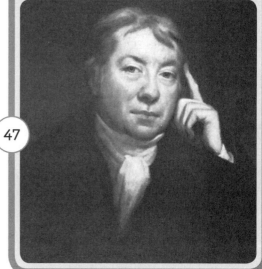

47

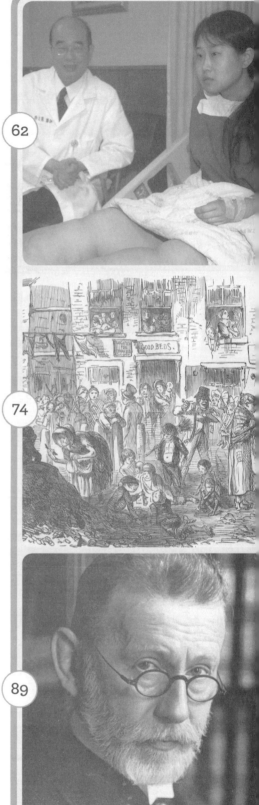

62

74

89

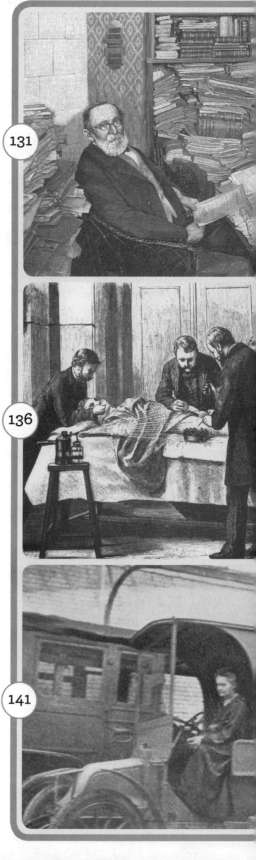

131

136

141

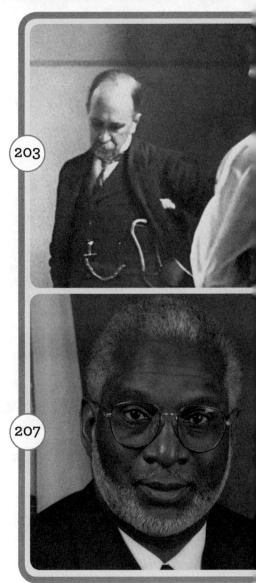

203

207

INTRODUCTION

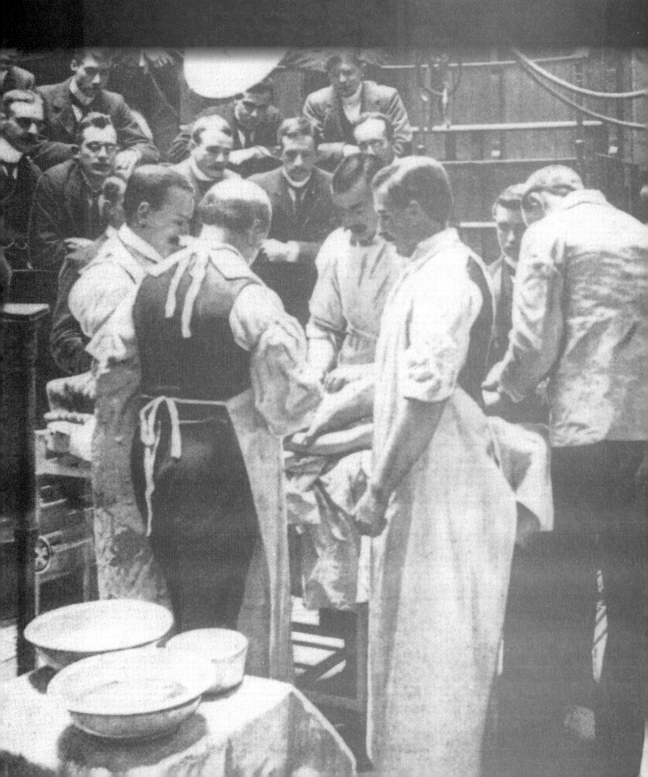

The history of medicine could be seen as a millennia-long progression from superstition to enlightenment. Although such a characterization might even be true in the broadest strokes, it would be a significant oversimplification of the fascinating story of the development of medical knowledge. In fact, remarkably sophisticated medicine was being practiced in some societies many centuries BCE, and some recent scientific discoveries have served to validate the efficacy of treatments once dismissed as old wives' tales.

What is unquestionably true is that the history of medicine has seen a steady progression in scientific knowledge of how the human body works, which has led to amazing advances in understanding the causes of disease as well as how to treat and prevent disease. In some cases, these advances have even led to the complete eradication of historically devastating diseases. The history of medicine is also very much the history of specific individuals who have made discoveries and advances relating to human anatomy and physiology, as well as those who have changed the practice of medicine through introducing new treatments and new policies. This book will introduce many of those individuals and will explore the ideas and practice of medicine from prehistory to the present day.

Medicine's story begins before the time of recorded history, with fossil remains of early humans showing evidence of healed bones and wounds and of scars from primitive surgery, perhaps performed to allow evil spirits to escape from the body. The earliest written record of the practice of medicine is in Hammurabi's code, an extensive code of laws written in Mesopotamia between 1792 and 1750 BCE. One section of the code is devoted to explaining laws on payments due for successful treatments and penalties for doctors who cause harm in the course of making incisions, removing tumours, and healing broken bones and other injuries. Papyri from ancient Egypt include entire treatises on the proper treatment of diseases using ointments, medications, and surgeries, with instructions for appropriate incantations to accompany each form of treatment.

Medicine was comparatively advanced in the early civilizations of Asia. Treatises on medical practice in India described some 1,120 different diseases and explained the use of hundreds of medicinal plants, minerals, and animal products. Surgical techniques were extremely advanced, including the removal of tumours and bladder stones, as well as cataracts. Chinese physicians also knew and used more than 1,000 different herbal, mineral, and animal products for the treatment of disease. The practice of acupuncture, designed to balance the distribution of yin and yang in the body, was widely used in ancient Chinese medicine.

Doctors performing surgery in London in the early 1900s. Buyenlarge/Archive Photos/Getty Images

Most of these early civilizations had strict religious prohibition against the mutilation of the dead, limiting the ability of early practitioners to study the parts of the human anatomy or to understand the workings of the body. Most treatments were no doubt discovered largely by trial and error, and by the time of their codification into medical texts, such as the ancient Egyptian papyri, the majority of the world's treatments for disease had been discovered. The theories of how and why these treatments worked, however, bear little resemblance to what is known today.

The Greek physician Hippocrates (c. 460 BCE–c. 375 BCE) has been referred to as the father of medicine because he is believed to have been the first to assert that diseases were the result of natural, rather than supernatural, causes. His legacy is also carried on today in the form of the Hippocratic oath, a code of high ethical conduct for physicians. Hippocrates—or others writing in his name—left extensive treatises detailing observations on disease and methods of healing. He was also famed as a teacher imparting his ideas to an entire generation of Greek physicians. For the next several centuries, Greek medicine was acknowledged to be the most advanced, and it was carried on through the medical school established in Alexandria, as well as by Greek-trained physicians during the Roman Empire.

After the fall of the Roman Empire, medical knowledge in Europe was largely maintained in the monasteries, both through the translation and transcription of classical medical texts and through the hospitals associated with many monasteries and convents. In the Islamic empire, extending from Persia across Northern Africa to Spain, physicians experimented in the field of chemistry, developing new techniques for purifying substances as well as discovering new medicines. In fact, many drugs that are in use today were originally developed by medieval Arabic scientists. Medical schools flourished in Cairo, Baghdad, and Córdoba, and textbooks written at these universities continued to be used well into the Middle Ages.

By the 14th and 15th centuries, the Renaissance brought a new enthusiasm for the advancement of knowledge through direct observation and experimentation, as opposed to following traditional teachings. Dissection of cadavers allowed for a much more precise knowledge of human anatomy and physiology. Italian physician Giralomo Fracastoro even advanced a theory in 1546 that the transmission of disease occurred through imperceptible particles in the air or through direct contact. Fracastoro's observations predated Louis Pasteur's actual discovery of such particles by more than 300 years. In the 1600s, British physician William Harvey published two landmark books describing his experiments and conclusions on the circulation of blood and the generation of life. Thus, medicine was beginning to adopt a scientific basis, a departure from the historical reliance on simple observation and theory. The invention of the microscope in the 17th century and of the stethoscope at the end of the 18th century contributed substantially to the advance of knowledge about the inner workings of the body.

Improvements in the understanding of the human body also began to influence the actual practice of healing the sick. Equally important in advancing medical practice was the openness to experimentation and observation. The discovery of an effective method of preventing smallpox by vaccination was one of the most significant medical advances of the 18th century, even though an understanding of the mechanism of immune response and the discovery of viruses were still a century or more away. Similarly, a British naval surgeon was able to eradicate scurvy among British sailors by recommending the addition of citrus fruits to their diet. The discovery of vitamin C, however, did not occur until the early 20th century.

In the 19th century, scientists began to look even deeper into human physiology, with one of the most important advances being the identification in the middle of the century of the cell as the centre of pathological changes causing the symptoms and effects of a variety of diseases. Equally influential was the confirmation by Louis Pasteur of germ theory – the idea that specific diseases are caused by specific microorganisms. Pasteur also made several other significant discoveries in the fields of epidemiology and immunology, including the creation of the first vaccine against rabies. Pasteur

was one of the most important figures in any century in the history of medical advances, despite the fact that he was a chemist and not a physician. His work influenced many other medical researchers, encouraging them to search for the specific bacteria responsible for a wide variety of diseases, including tuberculosis and cholera.

A practical impact of Pasteur's work was the work of Joseph Lister, who used the germ theory to develop and promote the importance of antiseptic barriers during surgeries and childbirth, leading to a dramatic decrease in death due to infections. Another innovation of the 19th century was the use of anesthesia during surgery. Pioneered by physicians in the United States, the practice was quickly adopted by surgeons in Europe, allowing for not only greater comfort on the part of the patient but also the possibility of longer and more complex surgeries.

The 19th century was also the age of imperialism in Europe. As Europeans took control of huge swaths of Africa, South America, and Asia, they were exposed to new tropical diseases. Wars of conquest and competition between the European powers also spread disease. English physicians demonstrated that mosquitoes were the means of transmission for tropical diseases such as malaria and yellow fever, and they developed measures to prevent infection. The Crimean War between Britain and Russia in 1853–56 also led to a new phase in the practice of medicine—the use of skilled, trained nurses in hospital care. This development was introduced by the work of Florence Nightingale and her recruits.

At the end of the century, another woman was also making a major contribution to medical history. In 1898, Marie Curie and her husband, Pierre, discovered and isolated radium. After her husband's early death, Marie Curie continued her research into the medical applications of radioactive substances, a field that revolutionized medicine in the 20th century. In fact, it was only during the 20th century that many of the advances taken for granted in medicine today were discovered. Major developments during this period included the introduction of antibiotics and the near eradication of common diseases through widespread vaccination.

In 1910 scientists for the first time isolated a chemical substance that was effective against a specific disease-causing bacterium. The organism was the bacterium that causes syphilis, and the discovery of the substance led to the development of a cure for the disease. Other antibacterial agents quickly followed, with the most dramatic being the discovery of penicillin in 1928 and its development as an antibiotic over the next decade. Penicillin was effective against a wide variety of infections, which led to the risk of infectious agents becoming resistant to it as physicians prescribed it freely. In the last half of the 20th century, a variety of other antibiotic agents allowed for more discriminate use, but the battle between antibiotic-resistant forms

of disease and the development of new antibiotics to treat them continues as an important issue in medical practice today.

During the same period when penicillin was developed, rapid advances were also being made in the creation of vaccines to prevent disease. Armies were vaccinated against typhoid and tetanus, diseases that had previously been as dangerous to the troops as battle deaths. An effective vaccine against diphtheria was developed in the 1920s, and by the 1960s had virtually wiped out the disease in countries where childhood vaccination was the norm. A vaccine for pertussis, or whooping cough, followed in the 1940s, and today most children in developed countries receive a combined DPT (diphtheria, pertussis, tetanus) injection in infancy.

Although the battle against bacterial diseases has been largely successful on two fronts—both treatment and prevention—viruses pose a different problem. Antibiotics are not effective against viral diseases, and scientists had little understanding of viruses until well into the 1930s. But as scientists were able to isolate and study viruses, vaccines began to be introduced. Perhaps the most important was the development of a vaccine against polio, introduced in the 1950s. Polio, or poliomyelitis, is a disease that most often affects children and can lead to lifelong paralysis. Although the most severe outcomes affected only a small portion of those infected, it was a constant worry for parents. Today polio is virtually unknown other than in isolated pockets of India and some countries in Africa. Public health officials believe it would be possible to eliminate the poliovirus entirely, as was done with smallpox, with concerted vaccination efforts in those areas where the disease still persists.

Other vaccines that also became available in the 20th century included several for common childhood diseases, including measles, mumps, chickenpox, and German measles (rubella). Today, most children never contract these diseases, which affected virtually every child only half a century earlier.

Another development of the 20th century was the understanding of the role of hormones in disease, allowing for effective management and treatment of diabetes by use of insulin, cortisone for rheumatoid arthritis, and hypothyroidism by injections of the thyroid hormone. An understanding of the role of hormones also allowed for the development of the birth control pill, by adjusting the levels of estrogen and progesterone to prevent ovulation and fertilization. Other diseases were found to be tied not to a deficiency in specific hormones, but to deficiencies in another 20th-century discovery—vitamins.

Today, the most common causes of death in previous centuries have nearly all been conquered or brought under control. Significant progress also has been made against human immunodeficiency virus (HIV), which causes AIDS. In addition, progress is being made in the treatment of cancer using radiation, chemotherapy, and surgery. A vaccine has even been introduced for cervical cancer. Cancer is now the second leading cause of death in most Western countries, following heart disease, partly because the population is now living longer rather than dying from other diseases at an early age.

Many medical practitioners today, particularly in primary practice and public health, focus not on illness, but on wellness. Obesity is now seen as one of the most important health threats, and lifestyle changes are the first line of defense for preventing diseases from adult-onset diabetes to heart disease. An understanding of environmental factors has also led to significant decreases in some cancers, notably lung cancer. The impact of stress hormones on health and on the immune system is also becoming better understood. The recommendations for healthy diet, rest, and fresh air promoted by Hippocrates and other early physicians remain sound medical advice today.

In laboratories of the 21st century, scientists at the frontiers of medical research are probing the human genome, exploring whether nerves can be regenerated to reverse paralysis, experimenting with genetically engineered drugs, and exploring the science of aging. Much of this work would have once been considered science fiction. Thus, the history of medicine, which began millennia ago, continues to be written by today's scientists and practitioners.

CHAPTER 1

ANCIENT MEDICINE AND ITS PRACTITIONERS

Medicine has been practiced in various ways throughout history. In primitive societies, the art of healing was an experimental process, guided in large part by trial and error. Many diseases were believed to have been brought upon humans by demons and other supernatural phenomena. Thus, much of the early art of healing dealt with intangible elements of human culture. Over time, however, as more became known about human disease and as the practice of medicine was gradually refined, systems of medicine embedded in folklore were surmounted by systems grounded in the scientific study of basic human anatomy and physiology (the study of the functioning of living organisms, animal or plant, and of the functioning of their constituent tissues or cells). This shift—heralded by the emergence of Western, or conventional, medicine—marked a major turning point in the history of medicine. Western medicine has since become the standard against which all other forms of medicine are measured for their ability to diagnose and treat human disease. Despite its dominance in the West, however, conventional medicine is not the most widely practiced form of medicine in the world today. Rather, various forms of traditional medicine, with origins in places such as Asia and Latin America, are the primary means of healing for the majority of the modern world's population.

The practitioners of medicine—the healers—have played a fundamental role in guiding the course of medicine over time. Ancient healers relied heavily on harvesting herbs and other natural products for the treatment of general conditions such as fever and gastrointestinal illness. Some of these early healers also experimented with rudimentary techniques for surgery and began to develop tools and approaches to correct physical conditions such as curvature of the spine. In the Renaissance and Enlightenment eras, physicians in the West learned of remedies used by practitioners of traditional medicine in Asia and the New World. In this way, knowledge of herbal cures from different regions of the world spread globally. The physicians of these eras also often recorded and published their observations of disease, which led to the discovery of new diseases and disorders and to better understanding of the causes of illness.

Medicine today is a reflection of the history of its practice and its practitioners. Over the course of time, approaches to the diagnosis and treatment of disease became subdivided into specialties, with physicians often focusing on specific organs or body systems. In the 20th century, the emergence of fields from immunology to endocrinology to oncology enabled medical students to narrow their academic studies and thereby tailor their expertise within a single area of practice. As a result, there occurred substantial and rapid progress in the scientific and medical understanding of health and disease. In the 21st century, continued advance in not only scientific knowledge but also in the training of nurses, scientists, and physicians has fueled the perpetual improvement of medicine and the art of healing.

PRIMITIVE MEDICINE AND FOLKLORE

Unwritten history is not easy to interpret, and, although much may be learned from a study of the drawings, bony remains, and surgical tools of early humans, it is difficult to reconstruct mental attitudes toward the problems of disease and death. It seems probable that humans, as soon as they had reached the stage of reasoning, discovered, by the process of trial and error, which plants might be used as foods, which of them were poisonous, and which of them had some medicinal value. Folk medicine or domestic medicine, consisting largely of the use of vegetable products, or herbs, originated in this fashion and still persists.

But that is not the whole story. Humans did not at first regard death and disease as natural phenomena. Common maladies, such as colds or constipation, were accepted as part of existence and dealt with by means of such herbal remedies as were available. Serious and disabling diseases, however, were placed in a very different category. These were of supernatural origin. They might be the result of a spell cast upon the victim by some enemy, visitation by a malevolent

MEDICINE MAN

The term medicine man *is used to describe a member of an indigenous society who is knowledgeable about the magical and chemical potencies of various substances (medicines) and skilled in the rituals through which they are administered. The term has been used most widely in the context of American Indian cultures but is applicable to many others as well. Despite the term's nomenclature, women perform this function in many societies.*

Traditionally, medicine people are called upon to prevent or heal the physical and mental illnesses of individuals as well as the social ruptures that occur when murders and other calamitous events take place within a community. Some medicine men and women undergo rigorous initiation to gain supernormal powers, while others become experts through apprenticeships; many complete a combination of these processes.

The medicine person commonly carries a kit of objects—feathers of particular birds, suggestively shaped or marked stones, pollen, hallucinogenic or medicinal plants, and other items—that are associated with healing. In some cases these materials are considered to have been drawn out of the body of the practitioner at his or her initiation to the healer's arts. Correspondingly, the work of healing often involves the extraction of offending substances from the patient's body by sucking, pulling, or other means. In some cases an object must be physically removed from the patient (e.g., the healer removes a projectile from a wound). In cases where the nature of the offending substance is metaphysical, however, the healing ritual focuses on achieving mental and spiritual health. In such cases a symbolic object may be "removed" from the patient by sleight of hand.

Because traditional indigenous belief systems often attribute illness and other distressing situations to the activities of witches or sorcerers, the term witch doctor, *denoting a person who diagnoses and treats such conditions, was coined by 18th-century Western observers. By the late 20th century the term was generally considered pejorative.*

demon, or the work of an offended god who had either projected some object—a dart, a stone, a worm—into the body of the victim or had abstracted something, usually the soul of the patient. The treatment then applied was to lure the errant soul back to its proper habitat within the body or to extract the evil intruder, be it dart or demon, by counterspells, incantations, potions, suction, or other means.

One curious method of providing the disease with means of escape from the body was by making a hole, 2.5 to 5 cm (1 to 2 inches) across, in the skull of the victim—the practice of trepanning, or trephining. Trepanned skulls of prehistoric date have been found in Britain, France, and other parts of Europe and in Peru. Many of them show evidence of healing and, presumably, of the patient's survival. The practice still exists among indigenous people in parts of Algeria, in Melanesia, and perhaps elsewhere, though it is becoming extinct.

Magic (as a mode of rationality or way of thinking that looks to invisible forces to influence events) and religion played a large part in the medicine of prehistoric or primitive humans. Administration of a vegetable drug or remedy by mouth was accompanied by incantations, dancing, grimaces, and all the tricks of the healer. Therefore, the first doctors, or "medicine men," were essentially sorcerers. The use of charms and talismans, still prevalent in modern times, is of ancient origin.

Apart from the treatment of wounds and broken bones, the folklore of medicine is probably the most ancient aspect of the art of healing, for primitive physicians showed their wisdom by treating the whole person, soul as well as body. Treatments and medicines that produced no physical effects on the body could nevertheless make a patient feel better when both medicine man and patient believed in their efficacy. This so-called placebo effect is applicable even in modern clinical medicine.

THE ANCIENT MIDDLE EAST AND EGYPT

The establishment of the calendar and the invention of writing marked the dawn of recorded history. The clues to early knowledge are scanty, consisting of clay tablets bearing cuneiform signs and seals that were used by physicians of ancient Mesopotamia. In the Louvre there is preserved a stone pillar on which is inscribed the Code of Hammurabi, who was a Babylonian king of the 18th century BCE. This code includes laws relating to the practice of medicine, and the penalties for failure were severe. For example, "If the doctor, in opening an abscess, shall kill the patient, his hands shall be cut off"; if, however, the patient was a slave, the doctor was simply obliged to supply another slave.

The Greek historian Herodotus stated that every Babylonian was an amateur physician, since it was the custom to lay the sick in the street so that anyone passing by might offer advice. Divination, from the inspection of the liver of a sacrificed animal, was widely practiced to foretell the course of a disease. Little else is known regarding Babylonian medicine, and the name of not a single physician has survived.

When the medicine of ancient Egypt is examined, the picture becomes clearer. The first physician to emerge is Imhotep, chief minister to King Djoser in the 3rd millennium BCE, who designed one of the earliest pyramids, the Step Pyramid at Ṣaqqārah, and who was later regarded as the Egyptian god of medicine and identified with the Greek god Asclepius.

Surer knowledge comes from the study of Egyptian papyri, especially the Edwin Smith and Ebers papyri discovered in the 19th century. The former is a surgical treatise on the treatment of wounds and other injuries, while the latter is a list of remedies. Dating from about 1550 BCE, the Ebers papyrus is one of the oldest known medical works. The scroll contains 700 magical formulas and folk remedies meant to cure afflictions

IMHOTEP

(b. 27th century BCE, Memphis, Egypt)

Imhotep (Greek: Imouthes) was a vizier, sage, architect, astrologer, and chief minister to Djoser (reigned 2630–2611 BCE), the second king of Egypt's third dynasty. Imhotep was later worshipped as the god of medicine in Egypt and in Greece, where he was identified with the Greek god of medicine, Asclepius. He is considered to have been the architect of the step pyramid built at the necropolis of Ṣaqqārah in the city of Memphis. The oldest extant monument of hewn stone known to the world, the pyramid consists of six steps and attains a height of 61 metres (200 feet).

Although no contemporary account has been found that refers to Imhotep as a practicing physician, ancient documents illustrating Egyptian society and medicine during the Old Kingdom (c. 2575–c. 2130 BCE) show that the chief magician of the pharaoh's court also frequently served as the nation's chief physician. Imhotep's reputation as the reigning genius of the time, his position in the court, his training as a scribe, and his becoming known as a medical demigod only 100 years after his death are strong indications that he must have been a physician of considerable skill.

Not until the Persian conquest of Egypt in 525 BCE was Imhotep elevated to the position of a full deity, replacing Nefertem in the great triad of Memphis, shared with his mythological parents Ptah, the creator of the universe, and Sekhmet, the goddess of war and pestilence. Imhotep's cult reached its zenith during Greco-Roman times, when his temples in Memphis and on the island of Philae (Arabic: Jazīrat Fīlah) in the Nile River were often crowded with sufferers who prayed and slept there with the conviction that the god would reveal remedies to them in their dreams. The only Egyptian mortal besides the 18th-dynasty sage and minister Amenhotep to attain the honour of total deification, Imhotep is still held in esteem by physicians who, like the eminent 19th-century British practitioner Sir William Osler, consider him "the first figure of a physician to stand out clearly from the mists of antiquity."

ranging from crocodile bite to toenail pain and to rid the house of such pests as flies, rats, and scorpions. It also includes a surprisingly accurate description of the circulatory system, noting the existence of blood vessels throughout the body and the heart's function as centre of the blood supply. The Ebers papyrus was acquired by George Maurice Ebers, a German Egyptologist and novelist, in 1873.

Contrary to what might be expected, the widespread practice of embalming the dead body did not stimulate study of human anatomy. The preservation of mummies has, however, revealed some of the diseases suffered at that time, including arthritis, tuberculosis of the bone, gout, tooth decay, bladder stones, and gallstones. There is evidence too of the parasitic disease schistosomiasis, which

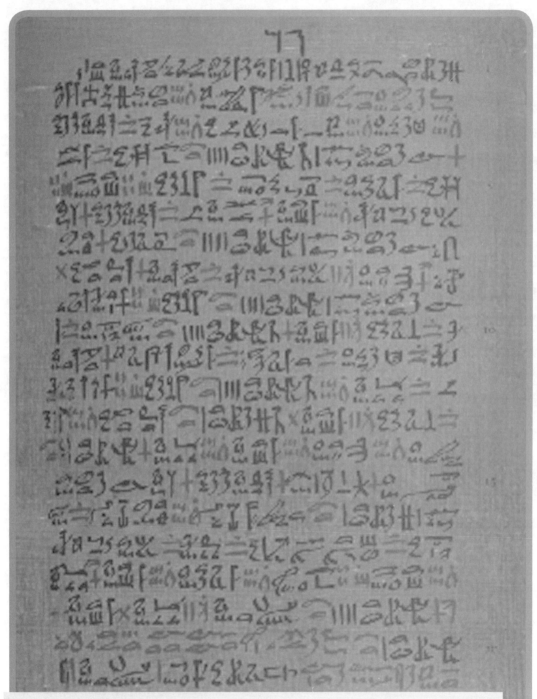

Prescription for asthma treatment on the Ebers papyrus. U.S. National Library of Medicine/ National Institutes of Health

remains a scourge still. There seems to have been no syphilis or rickets.

The search for information on ancient medicine leads naturally from the papyri of Egypt to Hebrew literature. Though the Bible contains little on the medical practices of Old Testament times, it is a mine of information on social and personal hygiene. The Jews were indeed pioneers in matters of public health.

TRADITIONAL MEDICINE AND SURGERY IN ASIA

Asia has a long history of medicine. Indeed, this region of the world is home to traditional practices of medicine, such as Āyurveda and traditional Chinese medicine, that originated thousands of years ago and are still widely used today. The history of traditional medicine in Asia is rooted in the ancient oral traditions of indigenous peoples. These traditions often are intertwined with folklore and tales, cultural beliefs, and local knowledge and skills. Much of this knowledge was first captured in writing many centuries ago in Asia. Among the oldest and most widely known medical writings from the region are India's Vedas, China's *Neijing*, and Japan's *Ishinhō*.

INDIA

Indian medicine has a long history. Its earliest concepts are set out in the sacred writings called the Vedas, especially in the metrical passages of the Atharvaveda, which may possibly date

as far back as the 2nd millennium BCE. According to a later writer, the system of medicine called Āyurveda was received by a certain Dhanvantari from Brahma, and Dhanvantari was deified as the god of medicine. In later times his status was gradually reduced, until he was credited with having been an earthly king who died of snakebite.

The period of Vedic medicine lasted until about 800 BCE. The Vedas are rich in magical practices for the treatment of diseases and in charms for the expulsion of the demons traditionally supposed to cause diseases. The chief conditions mentioned are fever (takman), cough, consumption, diarrhea, dropsy, abscesses, seizures, tumours, and skin diseases (including leprosy). The herbs recommended for treatment are numerous.

The golden age of Indian medicine, from 800 BCE until about 1000 CE, was marked especially by the production of the medical treatises known as the *Caraka-saṃhitā* and *Suśruta-saṃhitā*, attributed, respectively, to Caraka, a physician, and Suśruta, a surgeon. Estimates place the *Caraka-saṃhitā* in its present form as dating from the 1st century CE, although there were earlier versions. The *Suśruta-saṃhitā* probably originated in the last centuries BCE and had become fixed in its present form by the 7th century CE. Of somewhat lesser importance are the treatises attributed to Vagbhata. All later writings on Indian medicine were based on these works.

Because Hindus were prohibited by their religion from cutting the dead body, their knowledge of anatomy was limited. The *Suśruta-saṃhitā* recommends that a body be placed in a basket and sunk in a river for seven days. On its removal the parts could be easily separated without cutting. As a result of these crude methods, the emphasis in Hindu anatomy was given first to the bones and then to the muscles, ligaments, and joints. The nerves, blood vessels, and internal organs were very imperfectly known.

Hindus believed that the body contains three elementary substances, microcosmic representatives of the three divine universal forces, which they called spirit (air), phlegm, and bile (comparable to the humours of the Greeks). Health depends on the normal balance of these three elementary substances. The seven primary constituents of the body—blood, flesh, fat, bone, marrow, chyle, and semen—are produced by the action of the elementary substances. Semen was thought to be produced from all parts of the body and not from any individual part or organ.

Both Caraka and Suśruta state the existence of a large number of diseases (Suśruta says 1,120). Rough classifications of diseases are given. In all texts "fever," of which numerous types are described, is regarded as important. Phthisis (wasting disease, especially pulmonary tuberculosis) was apparently prevalent, and the Hindu physicians knew the symptoms of cases likely to terminate fatally. Smallpox was common, and it is probable that smallpox inoculation was practiced.

Hindu physicians employed all five senses in diagnosis. Hearing was used to distinguish the nature of the breathing, alteration in voice, and the grinding sound produced by the rubbing together of broken ends of bones. They appear to have had a good clinical sense, and their discourses on prognosis contain acute references to symptoms that have grave import. Magical beliefs still persisted, however, until late in the classical period. Thus, the prognosis could be affected by such fortuitous factors as the cleanliness of the messenger sent to fetch the physician, the nature of his conveyance, or the types of persons the physician met on his journey to the patient.

Dietetic treatment was important and preceded any medicinal treatment. Fats were much used, internally and externally. The most important methods of active treatment were referred to as the "five procedures": the administration of emetics, purgatives, water enemas, oil enemas, and sneezing powders. Inhalations were frequently administered, as were leeching, cupping, and bleeding.

The Indian materia medica (the body of knowledge of medicines) was extensive and consisted mainly of vegetable drugs, all of which were from indigenous plants. Caraka knew 500 medicinal plants, and Suśruta knew 760. But animal remedies (such as the milk of various animals, bones, gallstones) and minerals (such as sulfur, arsenic, lead, copper sulfate, gold) were also employed. The physicians collected and prepared their own vegetable drugs.

Among those that eventually appeared in Western pharmacopoeias were cardamom and cinnamon.

As a result of the strict religious beliefs of the Hindus, hygienic measures were important in treatment. Two meals a day were decreed, with indications of the nature of the diet, the amount of water to be drunk before and after the meal, and the use of condiments. Bathing and care of the skin were carefully prescribed, as were cleansing of the teeth with twigs from named trees, anointing of the body with oil, and the use of eyewashes.

In surgery, ancient Hindu medicine reached its zenith. Operations performed by Hindu surgeons included excision of tumours, incision and draining of abscesses, punctures to release fluid in the abdomen, extraction of foreign bodies, repair of anal fistulas, splinting of fractures, amputations, cesarean sections, and stitching of wounds.

A broad array of surgical instruments were used. According to Suśruta, the surgeon should be equipped with 20 sharp and 101 blunt instruments of various descriptions. The instruments were largely of steel. Alcohol seems to have been used as a narcotic during operations, and bleeding was stopped by hot oils and tar.

In two types of operations especially, the Hindus were outstanding. Stone in the bladder (vesical calculus) was common in ancient India, and the surgeons frequently removed the stones by lateral lithotomy. They also introduced plastic surgery. Amputation of the nose was one of the prescribed punishments for adultery, and repair was carried out by cutting from the patient's cheek or forehead a piece of tissue of the required size and shape and applying it to the stump of the nose. The results appear to have been tolerably satisfactory, and the modern operation is certainly derived indirectly from this ancient source. Hindu surgeons also operated on cataracts by couching, or displacing the lens to improve vision.

CHINA

The Chinese system of medicine is of great antiquity and is independent of any recorded external influences. According to legend, Emperor Huangdi (the Yellow Emperor) wrote the canon of internal medicine called the *Huangdi Neijing* (*The Yellow Emperor's Classic of Internal Medicine*) in the 3rd millennium BCE. But there is some evidence that in its present form it dates from no earlier than the 3rd century BCE. Most of the Chinese medical literature is founded on the *Neijing*, and it is still regarded as a great authority. Other famous works are the *Maijing* (known in the West as *The Pulse Classics*), composed about 300 CE, and the *Golden Mirror*, a compilation made about 1700 CE of medical writings of the Han dynasty (202 BCE–220 CE). European medicine began to obtain a footing in China early in the 19th century, but the native system is still widely practiced.

Basic to traditional Chinese medicine is the dualistic cosmic theory of the yin and the yang. The yang, the male principle, is active and light and is represented by the heavens; the yin, the female principle, is passive and dark and is represented by the earth. The human body, like matter in general, is made up of five elements: wood, fire, earth, metal, and water. With these are associated other groups of five, such as the five planets, the five conditions of the atmosphere, the five colours, and the five tones. Health, character, and the success of all political and private ventures are determined by the preponderance, at the time, of the yin or the yang; and the great aim of ancient Chinese medicine is to control their proportions in the body.

The teachings of the religious sects forbade the mutilation of the dead human body, and hence traditional anatomy rests on no sure scientific foundation. One of the most important writers on anatomy, Wang Qingren, gained his knowledge from the inspection of dog-torn children who had died in a plague epidemic in 1798 CE. Traditional Chinese anatomy is based on the cosmic system, which postulates the presence of such hypothetical structures as the 12 channels and the three so-called burning spaces. The body contains five organs (heart, lungs, liver, spleen, and kidneys), which store up but do not eliminate, and five viscera (such as the stomach, intestines, gallbladder, and bladder), which eliminate but do not store up. Each organ is associated with one of the planets, colours, tones, smells, and tastes. There are 365 bones and 365 joints in the body.

According to the physiology of traditional Chinese medicine, the blood vessels contain blood and air, in proportions varying with those of the yin and the yang. These two cosmic principles circulate in the 12 channels and control the blood vessels and hence the pulse. The Neijing says that "the blood current flows continuously in a circle and never stops. It may be compared to a circle without beginning or end." On this insubstantial evidence it has been claimed that the Chinese anticipated English physician William Harvey's 17th-century discovery of the circulation of the blood. Traditional Chinese pathology is also dependent on the theory of the yin and the yang. This led to an elaborate classification of diseases in which most of the types listed are without scientific foundation.

In diagnosis, detailed questions are asked about the history of the illness and about such things as the patient's taste, smell, and dreams. Conclusions are drawn from the quality of the voice, and note is made of the colour of the face and of the tongue. The most important part of the investigation, however, is the examination of the pulse. Wang Shuhe, who wrote The Pulse Classics, lived in the 3rd century BCE, and innumerable commentaries were written on his work. The pulse is examined in several places, at different times, and with varying degrees of pressure. The operation may take as long as three hours. It is often the only examination made, and it is used both for diagnosis and for prognosis. Not only are the diseased organs ascertained but the time of death or recovery may be foretold.

The Chinese materia medica has always been extensive and consists of vegetable, animal (including human), and mineral remedies. There were famous herbals from ancient times, but all these, to the number of about 1,000, were embodied by Li Shizhen in the compilation of *Bencao gangmu* (*Compendium of Materia Medica*) in the 16th century. This work, in 52 volumes, has been frequently revised and reprinted and is still authoritative. The use of drugs is mainly to restore the harmony of the yin and the yang and is also related to such matters as the five organs, the five planets, and the five colours. The art of prescribing is therefore complex.

Among the drugs taken over by Western medicine from the Chinese are rhubarb, iron (for anemia), castor oil, kaolin, aconite, camphor, and *Cannabis sativa* (Indian hemp). Chaulmoogra oil was used by the Chinese for leprosy from at least the 14th century. It was later introduced into Western medicine for this same purpose. The herb *ma huang* (*Ephedra vulgaris*) has been used in China for at least 4,000 years, and the isolation of the alkaloid ephedrine from it has greatly improved the Western treatment of asthma and similar conditions.

The most famous and expensive of Chinese remedies is ginseng. Western analysis has shown that it has diuretic and other properties but is of doubtful value. In recent years reserpine, the active principle of the Chinese plant *Rauwolfia,* has been isolated. It is now effectively used in the treatment of high blood pressure and some emotional and mental conditions.

Hydrotherapy is probably of Chinese origin, since cold baths were used for fevers as early as 180 BCE. The inoculation of smallpox matter, in order to produce a mild but immunizing attack of the disease, was practiced in China from ancient times and came to Europe about 1720. Another treatment is moxibustion, which consists of making a small, moistened cone (moxa) of powdered leaves of mugwort, or wormwood (*Artemisia* species), applying it to the skin, igniting it, and then crushing it into the blister so formed. Other substances are also used for the moxa. Dozens of these are sometimes applied at one sitting. The practice is often associated with acupuncture.

Acupuncture consists of the insertion into the skin and underlying tissues of a metal needle, either hot or cold. The theory is that the needle affects the distribution of the yin and the yang in the hypothetical channels and burning spaces of the body. The site of the insertion is chosen to affect a particular organ or organs. The practice of acupuncture dates from before 2500 BCE and is peculiarly Chinese. Little of practical importance has been added since that date, although there have been many well-known treatises on the subject.

A bronze model, *c.* 860 CE, shows the hundreds of specified points for the insertion of the needle. This was the forerunner of countless later models and diagrams. The needles used are 3 to 24 cm (about 1 to 9 inches) in length. They are often inserted with considerable force and after insertion may be agitated or screwed to the left or right. Acupuncture, often combined with moxibustion, is still widely used for many diseases, including fractures. People in the Western world have turned to acupuncturists for relief from pain and other symptoms. There is some speculation that the treatment may trigger the brain to release morphinelike substances called endorphins, which presumably reduce the feeling of pain and its concomitant emotions.

JAPAN

The most interesting features of Japanese medicine are the extent to which it was derivative and the rapidity with which, after a slow start, it became westernized and scientific. In the early pre-Christian Era disease was regarded as sent by the gods or produced by the influence of evil spirits. Treatment and prevention were based largely on religious practices, such as prayers, incantations, and exorcism. At a later date drugs and bloodletting were also employed.

Beginning in 608 CE, when young Japanese physicians were sent to China for a long period of study, Chinese influence on Japanese medicine was paramount. In 982, Tamba Yasuyori completed the 30-volume *Ishinhō*, the oldest Japanese medical work still extant. This work discusses diseases and their treatment, classified mainly according to the affected organs or parts. It is based entirely on older Chinese medical works,

with the yin and yang concept underlying the theory of disease causation.

In 1570 a 15-volume medical work was published by Menase Dōsan, who also wrote at least five other works. In the most significant of these, the *Keitekishū* (a manual of the practice of medicine, 1574), diseases—or sometimes merely symptoms—are classified and described in 51 groups. The work is unusual in that it includes a section on the diseases of old age. Another distinguished physician and teacher of the period, Nagata Tokuhun, whose important books were the *I-no-ben* (1585) and the *Baika mujinzo* (1611), held that the chief aim of the medical art was to support the natural force, and consequently that it was useless to persist with stereotyped methods of treatment unless the physician had the cooperation of the patient.

European medicine was introduced into Japan in the 16th century by Jesuit missionaries and again in the 17th century by Dutch physicians. Translations of European books on anatomy and internal medicine were made in the 18th century, and in 1836 an influential Japanese work on physiology appeared. In 1857 a group of Dutch-trained Japanese physicians founded a medical school in Edo (later Tokyo) that is regarded as the beginning of the medical faculty of the Imperial University of Tokyo.

During the last third of the 18th century it became government policy to westernize Japanese medicine, and great progress was made in the foundation of medical schools and the encouragement of research. Important medical break-throughs by the Japanese followed, among them the discovery of the plague bacillus in 1894, the discovery of a dysentery bacillus in 1897, the isolation of adrenaline (epinephrine) in crystalline form in 1901, and the first experimental production of a tar-induced cancer in 1918.

THE ROOTS OF WESTERN MEDICINE

The rise of Western medicine began in early Greece and gained support in the subsequent Hellenistic and Roman periods. The first form of medicine based exclusively on science was actually borne from the minds of Greek philosophers, who encouraged reason and consideration of natural forces over acceptance of the unknown. Thus, in ancient Greece, scientific theory, grounded largely in philosophical study, overtook the notion of healing as the dominion of the supernatural realm.

EARLY GREECE

The transition from magic to science was a gradual process that lasted for centuries, and there is little doubt that ancient Greece inherited much from Babylonia and Egypt, and even India and China. Twentieth-century readers of the Homeric tales the *Iliad* and the *Odyssey* may well be bewildered by the narrow distinction between gods and men among the characters and between historical fact and poetic fancy in the story. Two characters,

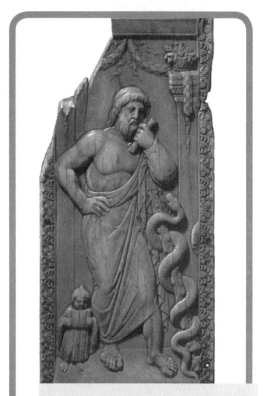

Asclepius, from an ivory diptych, 5th century AD; in the Liverpool City Museum, England. The Bridgeman Art Library/Art Resource, New York

the military surgeons Podaleirius and Machaon, are said to have been sons of Asclepius, the god of medicine. The divine Asclepius may have originated in a human Asclepius who lived about 1200 BCE and is said to have performed many miracles of healing.

Asclepius was worshiped in hundreds of temples throughout Greece, the remains of which may still be seen at Epidaurus, Cos, Athens, and elsewhere. To these resorts, or hospitals, sick persons went for the healing ritual known as incubation, or temple sleep. They lay down to sleep in the dormitory, or *aba-ton*, and were visited in their dreams by Asclepius or by one of his priests, who gave advice. In the morning the patient often is said to have departed cured. There are at Epidaurus many inscriptions recording cures, though there is no mention of failures or deaths.

Diet, baths, and exercises played their part in the treatment, and it would appear that these temples were the prototype of modern health resorts. Situated in a peaceful spot, with gardens and fountains, each had its theatre for amusements and its stadium for athletic contests. The cult of incubation continued far into the Christian Era. In Greece, some of the Aegean islands, Sardinia, and Sicily, sick persons are still taken to spend a night in certain churches in the hope of a cure.

It was, however, the work of the early philosophers, rather than that of the priests of Asclepius, that impelled Greeks to refuse to be guided solely by supernatural influence and moved them to seek out for themselves the causes and reasons for the strange ways of nature. The 6th-century philosopher Pythagoras, whose chief discovery was the importance of numbers, also investigated the physics of sound, and his views influenced the medical thought of his time. In the 5th century BCE Empedocles set forth the view that the universe is composed of four elements—fire, air, earth, and water. This conception led to the doctrine of the four bodily humours: blood; phlegm; choler, or yellow bile; and melancholy,

or black bile. The maintenance of health was held to depend upon the harmony of the four humours.

HIPPOCRATES
(b. c. 460 BCE, island of Cos, Greece—d. c. 375, Larissa, Thessaly)

Ancient Greek physician Hippocrates lived during Greece's Classical period and is traditionally regarded as the father of medicine. It is difficult to isolate the facts of Hippocrates' life from the later tales told about him or to assess his medicine accurately in the face of centuries of reverence for him as the ideal physician. About 60 medical writings have survived that bear his name, most of which were not written by him. He has been revered for his ethical standards in medical practice, mainly for the Hippocratic oath, which, it is suspected, he did not write.

LIFE AND WORKS

It is known that while Hippocrates was alive, he was admired as a physician and teacher. His younger contemporary Plato referred to him twice. In the *Protagoras* Plato called Hippocrates "the Asclepiad of Cos" who taught students for fees, and he implied that Hippocrates was as well known as a physician as Polyclitus and Phidias were as sculptors. It is now widely accepted that an "Asclepiad" was not a temple priest or a member of a physicians' guild but instead was a physician belonging to a family that had produced well-known physicians for generations.

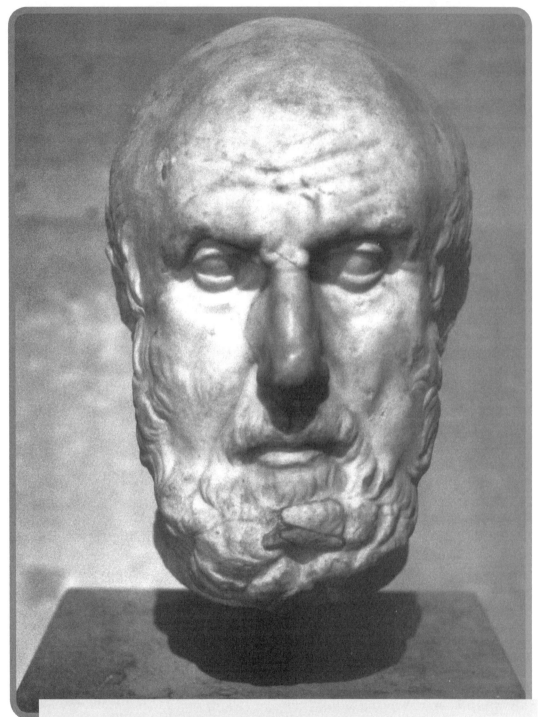

Hippocrates, undated bust. © Photos.com/Jupiterimages

Plato's second reference occurs in the *Phaedrus*, in which Hippocrates is referred to as a famous Asclepiad who had a philosophical approach to medicine.

Meno, a pupil of Aristotle, specifically stated in his history of medicine the views of Hippocrates on the causation of diseases, namely, that undigested residues were produced by unsuitable diet and that these residues excreted vapours, which passed into the body generally and produced diseases. Aristotle said that Hippocrates was called "the Great Physician" but that he was small in stature (*Politics*).

These are the only extant contemporary, or near-contemporary, references to Hippocrates. Five hundred years later, the Greek physician Soranus wrote a life of Hippocrates, but the contents of this and later lives were largely traditional or imaginative. Throughout his life Hippocrates appears to have traveled widely in Greece and Asia Minor practicing his art and teaching his pupils, and he presumably taught at the medical school at Cos quite frequently. His birth and death dates are traditional but may well be approximately accurate. Undoubtedly, Hippocrates was a historical figure, a great physician who exercised a permanent influence on the development of medicine and on the ideals and ethics of the physician.

Hippocrates' reputation, and myths about his life and his family, began to grow in the Hellenistic period, about a century after his death. During this period, the Museum of Alexandria in Egypt collected for its library literary material from preceding periods in celebration of the past greatness of Greece. So far as it can be inferred, the medical works that remained from the Classical period (among the earliest prose writings in Greek) were assembled as a group and called the works of Hippocrates (*Corpus Hippocraticum*). Linguists and physicians subsequently wrote commentaries on them, and, as a result, all the virtues of the Classical medical works were eventually attributed to Hippocrates and his personality constructed from them.

The virtues of the Hippocratic writings are many, and, although they are of varying lengths and literary quality, they are all simple and direct, earnest in their desire to help, and lacking in technical jargon and elaborate argument. The works show such different views and styles that they cannot be by one person, and some were clearly written in later periods. Yet all the works of the *Corpus* share basic assumptions about how the body works and what disease is, providing a sense of the substance and appeal of ancient Greek medicine as practiced by Hippocrates and other physicians of his era. Prominent among these attractive works are the *Epidemics*, which give annual records of weather and associated diseases, along with individual case histories and records of treatment, collected from cities in northern Greece. Diagnosis and prognosis are frequent subjects. Other treatises explain how to set fractures and treat wounds, feed and comfort patients, and take care of the body to avoid illness. Treatises called *Diseases* deal with serious illnesses, proceeding from the head to the feet, giving symptoms, prognoses, and treatments. There are works on diseases of women, childbirth, and pediatrics. Prescribed medications, other than foods and local salves, are generally purgatives to rid the body of the noxious substances thought to cause disease. Some works argue that medicine is indeed a science, with firm principles and methods, although explicit medical theory is very rare. The medicine depends on a mythology of how the body works and how its inner organs are connected. The myth is laboriously constructed from experience, but it must be remembered that there was neither systematic research nor dissection of human beings in Hippocrates' time. Hence, while much of the writing seems wise and correct, there are large areas where much is unknown.

The Embassy, a fictional work that connects Hippocrates' family with critical events in the history of Cos and Greece, was included in the original collection of Hippocratic works in the Library of Alexandria. Over the next four centuries, *The Embassy* inspired other imaginative writings, including letters between Hippocrates and the Persian king and also the philosopher Democritus. Though obviously fiction, these works enhanced Hippocrates' reputation, providing the basis for later biographies and the traditional picture of Hippocrates as the father of medicine. Still other works were added to the Hippocratic *Corpus* between its first collection and its first scholarly edition around the beginning of the 2nd century CE. Among them were the Hippocratic oath and other ethical writings that prescribe principles of behaviour for the physician.

INFLUENCE

Technical medical science developed in the Hellenistic period and after. Surgery, pharmacy, and anatomy advanced; physiology became the subject of serious speculation; and philosophic criticism improved the logic of medical theories. Competing schools in medicine (first Empiricism and later Rationalism) claimed Hippocrates as the origin and inspiration of their doctrines. In the 2nd century CE, the physician Galen of Pergamum developed his magnificent medical system, a synthesis of preceding work and his own additions that became the basis of European and Arabic medicine into the Renaissance. Galen was argumentative and long-winded, often abusive of contemporaries and earlier physicians, but at the same time, with exaggerated reverence that ignored five centuries of progress, he claimed that Hippocrates was the source of all that he himself knew and practiced. For later physicians, Hippocrates stood as the inspirational

HIPPOCRATIC OATH

The Hippocratic oath is an ethical code that comes from the works of Hippocrates (Corpus Hippocraticum). In addition to containing information on medical matters, the collection embodies a code of principles for the teachers of medicine and for their students. This code, or a fragment of it, has been handed down in various versions through generations of physicians as the Hippocratic oath. It has been used in the medical profession throughout the ages and is still read in the graduation ceremonies of many medical schools.

The oath dictates the obligations of the physician to students of medicine and the duties of pupil to teacher. In the oath, the physician pledges to prescribe only beneficial treatments, according to his abilities and judgment; to refrain from causing harm or hurt; and to live an exemplary personal and professional life.

The text of the Hippocratic oath (c. 400 BCE) provided here is a translation from Greek by Francis Adams (1849). It is considered a classical version and differs from contemporary versions, which are reviewed and revised frequently to fit with changes in modern medical practice.

I swear by Apollo the physician, and Aesculapius, and Health, and All-heal, and all the gods and goddesses, that, according to my ability and judgment, I will keep this Oath and this stipulation—to reckon him who taught me this Art equally dear to me as my parents, to share my substance with him, and relieve his necessities if required; to look upon his offspring in the same footing as my own brothers, and to teach them this Art, if they shall wish to learn it, without fee or stipulation; and that by precept, lecture, and every other mode of instruction, I will impart a knowledge of the Art to my own sons, and those of my teachers, and to disciples bound by a stipulation and oath according to the law of medicine, but to none others. I will follow that system of regimen which, according to my ability and judgment, I consider for the benefit of my patients, and abstain from whatever is deleterious and mischievous. I will give no deadly medicine to any one if asked, nor suggest any such counsel; and in like manner I will not give to a woman a pessary to produce abortion. With purity and with holiness I will pass my life and practice my Art. I will not cut persons laboring under the stone, but will leave this to be done by men who are practitioners of this work. Into whatever houses I enter, I will go into them for the benefit of the sick, and will abstain from every voluntary act of mischief and corruption; and, further from the seduction of females or males, of freemen and slaves. Whatever, in connection with my professional practice or not, in connection with it, I see or hear, in the life of men, which ought not to be spoken of abroad, I will not divulge, as reckoning that all such should be kept secret. While I continue to keep this Oath unviolated, may it be granted to me to enjoy life and the practice of the art, respected by all men, in all times! But should I trespass and violate this Oath, may the reverse be my lot!

source, while the more difficult Galen offered the substantial details.

As time went on, reverence for the past had to contend with new notions of scientific method and new discoveries. In the process, Galen's authority was undone, but Hippocrates' eminence as father of medicine remained. Scientific progress in fields such as anatomy, chemistry, microbiology, and microscopy, especially beginning in the 16th and 17th centuries, demanded that Galen's medicine be criticized and revised part by part. Arguments against Galenic medicine were often more effective when they were presented as returns to true Hippocratic medicine. New scientific methodology argued for a return to observation and study of nature, abandoning bookish authority. The simple and direct writings of the Hippocratic Collection read well as sample empirical texts that eschewed dogma. By the late 19th century, Galen was irrelevant to medical practice, and general knowledge of Hippocratic medical writings was beginning to fade. However, today Hippocrates still continues to represent the humane, ethical aspects of the medical profession. A number of idealized images of Hippocrates have survived from antiquity, but none that seems to derive from a contemporary portrait.

HELLENISTIC AND ROMAN MEDICINE

In the 4th century BCE the work of Aristotle, regarded as the first great biologist, was of inestimable value to medicine. A pupil of Plato at Athens and tutor to Alexander the Great, Aristotle studied the entire world of living things. He laid what can be identified as the foundations of comparative anatomy and embryology, and his views influenced scientific thinking for the next 2,000 years.

After the time of Aristotle, the centre of Greek culture shifted to Alexandria, where a famous medical school was established in about 300 BCE. There, the two best medical teachers were Herophilus, whose treatise on anatomy may have been the first of its kind, and Erasistratus, regarded by some as the founder of physiology. Erasistratus noted the difference between sensory and motor nerves but thought that the nerves were hollow tubes containing fluid and that air entered the lungs and heart and was carried through the body in the arteries. Alexandria continued as a centre of medical teaching even after the Roman Empire had attained supremacy over the Greek world, and medical knowledge remained predominantly Greek.

Asclepiades of Bithynia (born 124 BCE) differed from Hippocrates in that he denied the healing power of nature and insisted that disease should be treated safely, speedily, and agreeably. An opponent of the humoral theory, he drew upon the atomic theory of the 5th-century Greek philosopher Democritus in advocating a doctrine of *strictum et laxum*—the attribution of disease to the contracted or relaxed condition of the solid particles that he believed make up the body. To restore harmony among the particles and thus effect cures, Asclepiades used typically Greek remedies: massage, poultices, occasional tonics, fresh air, and corrective diet. He gave particular attention to mental disease, clearly distinguishing hallucinations from delusions. He released the insane from confinement in dark cellars and prescribed a regimen of occupational therapy, soothing music, soporifics (especially wine), and exercises to improve the attention and memory.

Asclepiades did much to win acceptance for Greek medicine in Rome. Aulus Cornelius Celsus, the Roman nobleman who wrote *De medicina* about 30 CE, gave a classic account of Greek medicine of the time, including descriptions of elaborate surgical operations. His book, overlooked in his day, enjoyed a wide reputation during the Renaissance.

During the early centuries of the Christian Era, Greek doctors thronged to Rome. The most illustrious of them was Galen, who began practicing there in 161 CE. He acknowledged his debt to Hippocrates and followed the Hippocratic method, accepting the doctrine of the humours. He laid stress on the value of anatomy, and he virtually founded experimental physiology. Galen recognized that the arteries contain blood and not merely air. He showed how the heart sets the blood in motion in an ebb and flow fashion, but he had no idea that the blood circulates. Dissection of the human body was at that time illegal, so that he was forced to base his knowledge upon the examination of animals, particularly apes. A voluminous writer who stated his views forcibly and with confidence, he remained for centuries the undisputed authority from whom no one dared to differ.

Another influential physician of the 2nd century CE was Soranus of Ephesus, who wrote authoritatively on childbirth, infant care, and women's diseases. An opponent of abortion, he advocated numerous means of contraception. He also described how to assist a difficult delivery by turning the fetus in the uterus (podalic version), a life-saving technique that was subsequently lost sight of until it was revived in the 16th century.

Although the contribution of Rome to the practice of medicine was negligible compared with that of Greece, in matters of public health the Romans set the world a great example. The city of Rome had an unrivaled water supply. Gymnasiums and public baths were provided, and there was even domestic sanitation and adequate disposal of sewage. The army had its medical officers, public physicians were appointed to attend the poor, and hospitals were built. A Roman hospital excavated near Düsseldorf, Ger., was found to be strikingly modern in design.

PUBLIC BATHS

Soaking the body in water or some other aqueous matter such as mud, steam, or milk may have cleanliness or curative purposes and may carry religious, mystical, or other meaning. The bath as an institution has a long history. Writings from ancient biblical and other sources mention baths. Architectural remains from ancient Egypt indicate the existence of special bathrooms, and both vase paintings and restored ruins show that the Greeks of classical antiquity thought the bath important. Roman baths featuring a combination of steaming, cleaning, and massage appeared wherever the Romans made conquests. In Rome itself the aqueducts fed sumptuous baths such as those of Caracalla, which covered 28 acres (11 hectares).

By medieval times in Europe the luxurious baths of ancient Rome had given way to more primitive facilities that had purely curative or cleanliness purposes. Public baths were built as early as the 12th century. In the 14th and 15th centuries public bathhouses and garden baths or pools accommodated men and women together. In the 1600s many persons visited spas to take baths, sometimes remaining submerged for health purposes for days at a time.

Modern baths have taken many forms. In some cases they have combined features from many types of older baths, including the Turkish bath and the Oriental tub bath, or furo. In the 1900s public baths frequently took the place of domestic facilities. In later decades the medicinal bath using a special tub or pool developed separately from the home bathtub or shower stall. The medicinal bath may use special waters, such as carbonated or chemically treated waters, at high or low temperatures.

PEDANIUS DIOSCORIDES
(b. c. 40 CE, Anazarbus, Cilicia—d. c. 90)

Greek physician and pharmacologist Pedanius Dioscorides was known for his work *De materia medica*, which was the foremost classical source of modern botanical terminology and the leading pharmacological text for 16 centuries.

Dioscorides' travels as a surgeon with the armies of the Roman emperor Nero provided him an opportunity to study the features, distribution, and medicinal properties of many plants and minerals. Excellent descriptions of nearly 600 plants, including cannabis, colchicum, water hemlock, and peppermint, are contained in *De materia medica*. Written in five books around the year 77, this work deals with approximately 1,000 simple drugs.

The medicinal and dietetic value of animal derivatives such as milk and honey is described in the second book, and a synopsis of such chemical drugs as mercury (with directions for its preparation from cinnabar), arsenic (referred to as auripigmentum, the yellow arsenic sulfide), lead acetate, calcium hydrate, and copper oxide is found in the fifth book. He clearly refers to sleeping potions prepared from opium and mandragora as surgical anesthetics.

Although the work may be considered little more than a drug collector's manual by modern standards, the original Greek manuscript, which was copied in at least seven other languages, describes most drugs used in medical practice until modern times and served as the primary text of pharmacology until the end of the 15th century. Modern editions have been published in Greek (1906–14) and in English (1934).

GALEN OF PERGAMUM
(b. 129 CE, Pergamum, Mysia, Anatolia [now Bergama, Tur.]—d. *c.* 216)

Greek physician, writer, and philosopher Galen of Pergamum (Latin: Galenus) exercised a dominant influence on medical theory and practice in Europe from the Middle Ages until the mid-17th century. His authority in the Byzantine world and the Muslim Middle East was similarly long-lived.

Early Life and Training

The son of a wealthy architect, Galen was educated as a philosopher and man of letters. His hometown, Pergamum, was the site of a magnificent shrine of the healing god, Asclepius, that was visited by many distinguished figures of the Roman Empire for cures. When Galen was 16, he changed his career to that of medicine, which he studied at Pergamum, at Smyrna (modern İzmir, Tur.), and finally at Alexandria in Egypt, which was the greatest medical centre of the ancient

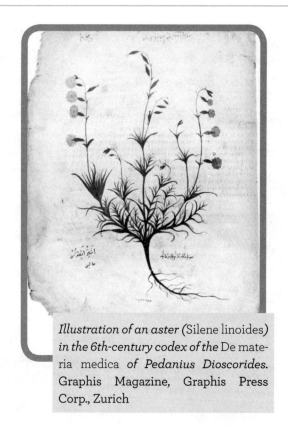

Illustration of an aster (Silene linoides) *in the 6th-century codex of the* De materia medica *of Pedanius Dioscorides.* Graphis Magazine, Graphis Press Corp., Zurich

world. After more than a decade of study, he returned in 157 CE to Pergamum, where he served as chief physician to the troop of gladiators maintained by the high priest of Asia.

In 162 the ambitious Galen moved to Rome. There he quickly rose in the medical profession owing to his public demonstrations of anatomy, his successes with rich and influential patients whom other doctors had pronounced incurable, his enormous learning, and the rhetorical skills he displayed in public debates. Galen's wealthy background, social contacts, and friendship with his old philosophy teacher Eudemus further enhanced his reputation as a philosopher and physician.

Galen abruptly ended his sojourn in the capital in 166. Although he claimed that the intolerable envy of his colleagues prompted his return to Pergamum, an impending plague in Rome was probably a more compelling reason. In 168–169, however, he was called by the joint emperors Lucius Verus and Marcus Aurelius to accompany them on a military campaign in northern Italy. After Verus's sudden death in 169, Galen returned to Rome, where he served Marcus Aurelius and the later emperors Commodus and Septimius Severus as a physician. Galen's final works were written after 207, which suggests that his Arab biographers were correct in their claim that he died at age 87, in 216/217.

Anatomical and Medical Studies

Galen regarded anatomy as the foundation of medical knowledge, and he frequently dissected and experimented on such lower animals as the Barbary ape (or African monkey), pigs, sheep, and goats. Galen's advocacy of dissection, both to improve surgical skills and for research purposes, formed part of his self-promotion, but there is no doubt that he was an accurate observer. He distinguished seven pairs of cranial nerves, described the valves of the heart, and observed the structural differences between arteries and veins. One of his most important demonstrations was that the arteries carry blood, not air, as had been taught for 400 years. Notable also were his vivisection experiments, such

as tying off the recurrent laryngeal nerve to show that the brain controls the voice, performing a series of transections of the spinal cord to establish the functions of the spinal nerves, and tying off the ureters to demonstrate kidney and bladder functions. Galen was seriously hampered by the prevailing social taboo against dissecting human corpses, however, and the inferences he made about human anatomy based on his dissections of animals often led him into errors. His anatomy of the uterus, for example, is largely that of the dog's.

Galen's physiology was a mixture of ideas taken from the philosophers Plato and Aristotle as well as from the physician Hippocrates, whom Galen revered as the fount of all medical learning. Galen viewed the body as consisting of three connected systems: the brain and nerves, which are responsible for sensation and thought; the heart and arteries, responsible for life-giving energy; and the liver and veins, responsible for nutrition and growth. According to Galen, blood is formed in the liver and is then carried by the veins to all parts of the body, where it is used up as nutriment or is transformed into flesh and other substances. A small amount of blood seeps through the lungs between the pulmonary artery and pulmonary veins, thereby becoming mixed with air, and then seeps from the right to the left ventricle of the heart through minute pores in the wall separating the two chambers. A small proportion of this blood is further refined in a network of nerves at the base of the skull (in reality found only

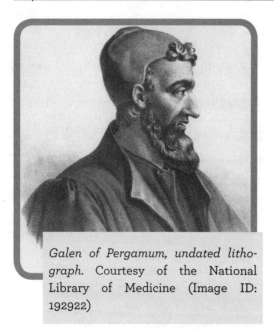

Galen of Pergamum, undated lithograph. Courtesy of the National Library of Medicine (Image ID: 192922)

conceptions, Galenic physiology became a powerful influence in medicine for the next 1,400 years.

Galen was both a universal genius and a prolific writer: about 300 titles of works by him are known, of which about 150 survive wholly or in part. He was perpetually inquisitive, even in areas remote from medicine, such as linguistics, and he was an important logician who wrote major studies of scientific method. Galen was also a skilled polemicist and an incorrigible publicist of his own genius, and these traits, combined with the enormous range of his writings, help to explain his subsequent fame and influence.

in ungulates) and the brain to make psychic pneuma, a subtle material that is the vehicle of sensation. Galen's physiological theory proved extremely seductive, and few possessed the skills needed to challenge it in succeeding centuries.

Building on earlier Hippocratic conceptions, Galen believed that human health requires an equilibrium between the four main bodily fluids, or humours— blood, yellow bile, black bile, and phlegm. Each of the humours is built up from the four elements and displays two of the four primary qualities: hot, cold, wet, and dry. Unlike Hippocrates, Galen argued that humoral imbalances can be located in specific organs, as well as in the body as a whole. This modification of the theory allowed doctors to make more precise diagnoses and to prescribe specific remedies to restore the body's balance. As a continuation of earlier Hippocratic

Galen's Influence

Galen's writings achieved wide circulation during his lifetime, and copies of some of his works survive that were written within a generation of his death. By 500 CE his works were being taught and summarized at Alexandria, and his theories were already crowding out those of others in the medical handbooks of the Byzantine world. Greek manuscripts began to be collected and translated by enlightened Arabs in the 9th century, and about 850 Ḥunayn ibn Isḥāq, an Arab physician at the court of Baghdad, prepared an annotated list of 129 works of Galen that he and his followers had translated from Greek into Arabic or Syriac. Learned medicine in the Arabic world thus became heavily based upon the commentary, exposition, and understanding of Galen.

Galen's influence was initially almost negligible in western Europe except for drug recipes, but from the late 11th century Ḥunayn's translations, commentaries on them by Arab physicians, and sometimes the original Greek writings themselves were translated into Latin. These Latin versions came to form the basis of medical education in the new medieval universities. From about 1490, Italian humanists felt the need to prepare new Latin versions of Galen directly from Greek manuscripts in order to free his texts from medieval preconceptions and misunderstandings. Galen's works were first printed in Greek in their entirety in 1525, and printings in Latin swiftly followed. These texts offered a different picture from that of the Middle Ages, one that emphasized Galen as a clinician, a diagnostician, and above all, an anatomist. His new followers stressed his methodical techniques of identifying and curing illness, his independent judgment, and his cautious empiricism. Galen's injunctions to investigate the body were eagerly followed, since physicians wished to repeat the experiments and observations that he had recorded. Paradoxically, this soon led to the overthrow of Galen's authority as an anatomist. In 1543 the Flemish physician Andreas Vesalius showed that Galen's anatomy of the body was more animal than human in some of its aspects, and it became clear that Galen and his medieval followers had made many errors. Galen's notions of physiology, by contrast, lasted for a further century, until the English physician William Harvey correctly explained the circulation of the blood. The renewal and then the overthrow of the Galenic tradition in the Renaissance had been an important element in the rise of modern science, however.

CHAPTER 2

MEDICINE IN THE MEDIEVAL AND RENAISSANCE ERAS

After the fall of Rome, learning was no longer held in high esteem, experiment was discouraged, and originality became a dangerous asset. During the early Middle Ages, medicine passed into the widely diverse hands of the Christian Church and Arab scholars. The Arabs, in their efforts to translate the works of the ancient Greeks, served a vital role in advancing science and medicine. Among the most remarkable physicians of the medieval Muslim world was Avicenna, noted for his influential and comprehensive medical writings.

In Europe, the Middle Ages was followed by the Renaissance, or "rebirth." During this period, the Arabic translations of early Greek works entered Europe and were used in universities across the region. As a result, much of European scholarship became anchored in Greek philosophy. And as the philosophical and scientific theories of the ancient Greeks became widely known, the understanding of disease by European physicians became increasingly grounded in science. Thus, the shadow of sin and repentance cast upon human disease by the church was shed. The ensuing scientific developments of the Renaissance proved fundamental in propelling Western medicine to the forefront of science and medical practice in the centuries that followed.

CHRISTIAN AND MUSLIM RESERVOIRS OF LEARNING

It is sometimes stated that the early Christian Church had an adverse effect upon medical progress. Disease was regarded as a punishment for sin, and such chastening demanded only prayer and repentance. Moreover, the human body was held sacred and dissection was forbidden. But the infinite care and nursing bestowed upon the sick under Christian auspices must outweigh any intolerance shown toward medicine in the early days.

TRANSLATORS AND SAINTS

Perhaps the greatest service rendered to medicine by the church was the preservation and transcription of the classical Greek medical manuscripts. These were translated into Latin in many medieval monasteries, and the Nestorian Christians (an Eastern church) established a school of translators to render the Greek texts into Arabic. This famous school, and also a great hospital, were located at Jundi Shāhpūr in southwest Persia, where the chief physician was Jurjīs ibn Bukhtīshū', the first of a dynasty of translators and physicians that lasted for six generations. A later translator of great renown was Ḥunayn ibn Isḥāq, whose translations were said to be worth their weight in gold.

About this time there appeared a number of saints whose names were associated with miraculous cures. Among the earliest of these were twin brothers, Cosmas and Damian, who suffered martyrdom (c. 303 CE) and who became the patron saints of medicine. Other saints were invoked as powerful healers of

ḤUNAYN IBN ISḤĀQ

(b. 808, al-Ḥīrah, near Baghdad, Iraq—d. 873, Baghdad)

Arab scholar Ḥunayn ibn Isḥāq (Latin: Johannitius) was known for his translations of Plato, Aristotle, Galen, Hippocrates, and the Neoplatonists, which made the significant sources of Greek thought and culture accessible to Arab philosophers and scientists.

Ḥunayn was a Nestorian Christian who studied medicine in Baghdad and became well versed in ancient Greek. He was appointed by Caliph al-Mutawakkil to the post of chief physician to the court, a position that he held for the rest of his life. He traveled to Syria, Palestine, and Egypt to gather ancient Greek manuscripts, and, from his translators' school in Baghdad, he and his students transmitted Arabic and (more frequently) Syriac versions of the classical Greek texts throughout the Islamic world. Especially important are his translations of Galen, most of the original Greek manuscripts of which are lost.

certain diseases, such as St. Vitus for chorea (or St. Vitus' dance) and St. Anthony for erysipelas (or St. Anthony's fire). The cult of these saints was widespread in medieval times, and a later cult, that of St. Roch for plague, was widespread during the plague-ridden years of the 14th century.

ARABIAN MEDICINE

A second reservoir of medical learning during those times was the great Muslim empire, which extended from Persia to Spain. Although it is customary to speak of Arabian medicine in describing this period (roughly, the 7th to the 14th century), not all of the physicians were Arabs. Nor, indeed, were they all Muslims: some were Jews, some Christians, and they were drawn from all parts of the empire. One of the earliest figures was al-Rāzī, a Persian born in the last half of the 9th century near modern Tehran. Of later date was Avicenna (980–1037), who has been called the prince of physicians and whose tomb at Hamadan has become a place of pilgrimage. Both were famous for writing influential medical texts.

The greatest contribution of Arabian medicine was in chemistry and in the knowledge and preparation of medicines. The chemists of that time were alchemists, and their pursuit was mainly a search for the philosopher's stone, which supposedly would turn common metals into gold. In the course of their experiments, however, numerous substances were named and characterized, and some were found to have medicinal value. Many drugs now in use are of Arab origin, as are such processes as distillation and sublimation.

At that period, and indeed throughout most historical times, surgery was considered inferior to medicine, and surgeons were held in low regard. The renowned Spanish surgeon Abū al-Qāsim (Albucasis), however, did much to raise the status of surgery in Córdoba, an important centre of commerce and culture with a hospital and medical school equal to those of Cairo and Baghdad. A careful and conservative practitioner, he wrote the first illustrated surgical text, which held wide influence in Europe for centuries.

Another great doctor of Córdoba, born in the 12th century, just as the sun of Arabian culture was setting there, was the Jewish philosopher Maimonides. Banished from the city because he would not become a Muslim, he eventually went to Cairo, where the law was more lenient and where he acquired a reputation so high that he became physician to Saladin, a Muslim sultan and the founder of the Ayyūbid dynasty. A few of his works, written in Hebrew, were eventually translated into Latin and printed.

AL-RĀZĪ
(b. c. 854, Rayy, Persia [now in Iran]—d. 925/935, Rayy)

Celebrated alchemist and Muslim philosopher al-Rāzī (Latin: Rhazes) is considered one of the greatest physicians of the Islamic world.

One tradition holds that al-Rāzī was already an alchemist before he gained his medical knowledge. After serving as chief physician in a Rayy hospital, he held a similar position in Baghdad for some time. Like many intellectuals in his day, he lived at various small courts under the patronage of minor rulers. With references to his Greek predecessors, al-Rāzī viewed himself as the Islamic version of Socrates in philosophy and of Hippocrates in medicine.

Al-Rāzī's two most significant medical works are the *Kitāb al-Manṣūrī*, which he composed for the Rayy ruler Manṣūr ibn Isḥaq and which became well known in the West in Gerard of Cremona's 12th-century Latin translation; and *Kitāb al-ḥāwī* (*Comprehensive Book*), in which he surveyed Greek, Syrian, and early Arabic medicine, as well as some Indian medical knowledge. Throughout his works he added his own considered judgment and his own medical experience as commentary. Among his numerous minor medical treatises is the famed, *De variolis et morbillis* (*A Treatise on the Smallpox and Measles*), which distinguishes between these two diseases and gives a clear description of both. It was translated into Latin, Byzantine Greek, and various modern languages.

The philosophical writings of al-Rāzī were neglected for centuries, and renewed appreciation of their importance did not occur until the 20th century. Although he claimed to be a follower of Plato, he consistently disagreed with such Arabic interpreters of Plato as al-Fārābī, Avicenna, and Averroës. He was probably acquainted with Arabic translations of the Greek atomist philosopher Democritus and pursued a similar tendency in his own atomic theory of the composition of matter. Among his other works, *The Spiritual Physick of Rhazes* is a popular ethical treatise and a major alchemical study.

AVICENNA
(b. 980, near Bukhara, Iran [now in Uzbekistan]—d. 1037, Hamadan)

Muslim physician Avicenna (Arabic: Ibn Sīnā) is the most famous and influential of the philosopher-scientists of the Islamic world. He was particularly noted for his contributions in the fields of Aristotelian philosophy and medicine. He composed the *Kitāb al-shifāʾ* (*Book of the Cure*), a vast philosophical and scientific encyclopaedia, and *Al-Qanun fi al-Tibb* (*The Canon of Medicine*), which is among the most famous books in the history of medicine. It was used at many medical schools—at Montpellier, France, as late as 1650—and reputedly is still used in the East.

Avicenna did not burst upon an empty Islamic intellectual stage. More than two centuries before him, it is believed that Muslim writer Ibn al-Muqaffaʿ, or possibly his son, had introduced Aristotelian logic to the Islamic world. Al-Kindī, the first Islamic Peripatetic (Aristotelian) philosopher, and Turkish polymath al-Fārābī, from whose book Avicenna would learn Aristotle's metaphysics, preceded him.

Of these luminaries, however, Avicenna remains by far the greatest.

Life and Education

According to Avicenna's personal account of his life, as communicated in the records of his longtime pupil al-Jūzjānī, he read and memorized the entire Qur'ān by age 10. The tutor Nātilī instructed the youth in elementary logic, and, having soon surpassed his teacher, Avicenna took to studying the Hellenistic authors on his own. By age 16, Avicenna turned to medicine, a discipline over which he claimed "easy" mastery. When the sultan of Bukhara fell ill with an ailment that baffled the court physicians, Avicenna was called to his bedside and cured him. In gratitude, the sultan opened the royal Sāmānid library to him, a fortuitous benevolence that introduced Avicenna to a veritable cornucopia of science and philosophy.

Avicenna began his prodigious writing career at age 21. Some 240 extant titles bear his name. They cross numerous fields, including mathematics, geometry, astronomy, physics, metaphysics, philology, music, and poetry. Often caught up in the tempestuous political and religious strife of the era, Avicenna's scholarship was unquestionably hampered by a need to remain on the move. At Eṣfahān, under 'Alā al-Dawla, he found the stability and security that had eluded him. If Avicenna could be said to have had any halcyon days, they occurred during

his time at Eṣfahān, where he was insulated from political intrigues and could hold his own scholars' court every Friday, discussing topics at will. In this salubrious climate Avicenna completed *Kitāb al-shifā'*, wrote *Dānish nāma-i 'alā'ī* (*Book of Knowledge*) and *Kitāb al-najāt* (*Book of Salvation*), and compiled new and more accurate astronomical tables.

While in the company of 'Alā al-Dawla, Avicenna fell ill with colic. He treated himself by employing the heroic measure of eight self-administered celery-seed enemas in one day. However, the preparation was either inadvertently or intentionally altered by an attendant to include five instead of the prescribed two measures of active ingredient. This caused ulceration of the intestines. Following up with mithridate (a mild opium remedy attributed to Mithradates VI Eupator, king of Pontus [120–63 BCE]), a slave attempted to poison Avicenna by surreptitiously adding a surfeit of opium. Weakened but indefatigable, he accompanied 'Alā al-Dawla on his march to Hamadan. On the way he took a severe turn for the worse, lingered for a while, and died in the holy month of Ramadan.

Influence in Medicine

Despite a general assessment favouring al-Rāzī's medical contributions, many physicians historically preferred Avicenna for his organization and clarity. Indeed, his influence over Europe's great medical schools extended well into the early modern period. Here, *The Canon of Medicine (Al-Qanun fi al-Tibb)* became the preeminent source, rather than al-Rāzī's *Kitāb al-ḥāwī (Comprehensive Book)*.

Avicenna's penchant for categorizing becomes immediately evident in the *Canon*, which is divided into five books. The first book contains four treatises, the first of which examines the four elements (earth, air, fire, and water) in light of Greek physician Galen of Pergamum's four humours (blood, phlegm, yellow bile, and black bile). The first treatise also includes anatomy. The second treatise examines etiology (cause) and symptoms, while the third covers hygiene, health and sickness, and death's inevitability. The fourth treatise is a therapeutic nosology (classification of disease) and a general overview of regimens and dietary treatments. Book II of the *Canon* is a "Materia Medica," Book III covers "Head-to-Toe Diseases," Book IV examines "Diseases That Are Not Specific to Certain Organs" (fevers and other systemic and humoral pathologies), and Book V presents "Compound Drugs" (e.g., theriacs, mithridates, electuaries, and cathartics). Books II and V each offer important compendia of about 760 simple and compound drugs that elaborate upon Galen's humoral pathology.

Unfortunately, Avicenna's original clinical records, intended as an appendix to the *Canon*, were lost, and only an Arabic text has survived in a Roman publication of 1593. Yet, he obviously practiced Greek physician Hippocrates' treatment of spinal deformities with reduction techniques, an approach that had been refined by Greek physician and surgeon Paul of Aegina. Reduction involved the use of pressure and traction to straighten or otherwise correct bone and joint deformities such as curvature of the spine. The techniques were not used again until French surgeon Jean-François Calot reintroduced the practice in 1896. Avicenna's suggestion of wine as a wound dressing was commonly employed in medieval Europe. He also described a condition known as "Persian fire" (anthrax), correctly correlated the sweet taste of urine to diabetes, and described the guinea worm.

MEDIEVAL AND RENAISSANCE EUROPE

Many important medical schools, including the famed university at Salerno in Italy, were established in Europe in the Middle Ages. Although many teachers of medicine in the medieval universities clung to the past, there were some who explored new lines of thought. One such individual was Italian physician Mondino dei Liucci, who was known for his public lectures in which he performed dissections of the human body. During the Renaissance, a period born in Italy in the 14th century, the new learning grew and expanded slowly. Influential in promoting its expansion were the Renaissance figures Belgian physician Andreas Vesalius and Italian surgeon and anatomist Hieronymus Fabricius ab Aquapendente.

SALERNO AND THE MEDICAL SCHOOLS

At about the same time that Arabian medicine flourished, the first organized medical school in Europe was established at Salerno, in southern Italy. Although the school of Salerno produced no brilliant genius and no startling discovery, it was the outstanding medical institution of its time and the parent of the great medieval schools soon to be founded at Montpellier and Paris, in France, and at Bologna and Padua, in Italy. Salerno drew scholars from near and far. Remarkably liberal in some of its views, Salerno admitted women as medical students. The school owed much to the enlightened Holy Roman emperor Frederick II, who decreed in 1221 that no one should practice medicine until he had been publicly approved by the masters of Salerno.

The Salernitan school also produced a literature of its own. The best-known work, of uncertain date and of composite authorship, was the *Regimen Sanitatis Salernitanum* (*Salernitan Guide to Health*). Written in verse, it has appeared in numerous editions and has been translated into many languages. Among its oft-quoted couplets is the following:

> *Use three physicians still, first Doctor Quiet,*
> *Next Doctor Merryman, and Doctor Diet.*

Salerno yielded its place as the premier medical school of Europe to Montpellier in about 1200. John of Gaddesden, the model for the "doctour of physick" in Chaucer's *Canterbury Tales*, was one of the English students there. That he relied upon astrology and upon the doctrine of the humours is evident from Chaucer's description:

> *Well could he guess the ascending of the star*
> *Wherein his patient's fortunes settled were.*
> *He knew the course of every malady,*
> *Were it of cold or heat or moist or dry.*

Medieval physicians analyzed symptoms, examined excreta, and made their diagnoses. Then they might prescribe diet, rest, sleep, exercise, or baths. Or they could administer emetics and purgatives or bleed the patient. Surgeons could treat fractures and dislocations, repair hernias, and perform amputations and a few other operations. Some of them prescribed opium, mandragora, or alcohol to deaden pain. Childbirth was left to midwives, who relied on folklore and tradition.

Great hospitals were established during the Middle Ages by religious foundations, and infirmaries were attached to abbeys, monasteries, priories, and convents. Doctors and nurses in these institutions were members of

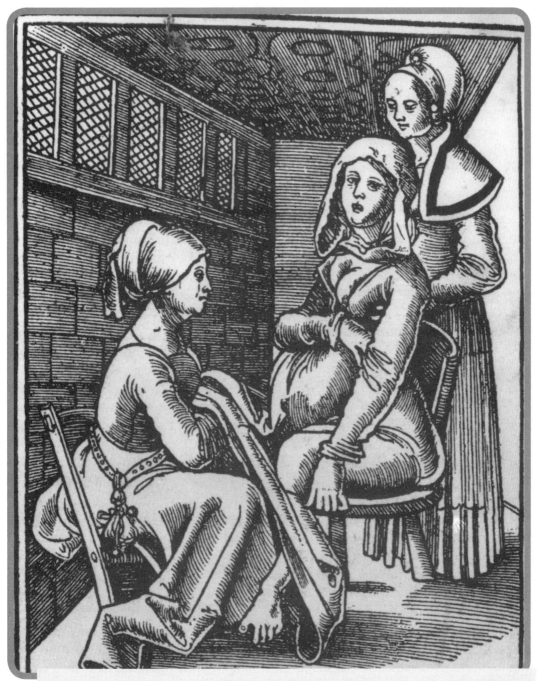

This 1513 illustration shows a midwife and friend attending to a woman giving birth at home. Hulton Archive/Getty Images

religious orders and combined spiritual with physical healing.

The Spread of New Learning

Two great 13th-century scholars who influenced medicine were Roger Bacon, an active observer and tireless experimenter, and Albertus Magnus, a distinguished philosopher and scientific writer. Also around this time Mondino dei Liucci taught at Bologna. Prohibitions against human dissection were slowly lifting, and Mondino performed his own dissections rather than following the customary procedure of entrusting the task to a menial. Although he perpetuated the errors of Galen, his *Anothomia*, published in 1316, was the first practical manual of anatomy. Foremost among the surgeons of the day was Guy de Chauliac, a physician to three popes at Avignon. His *Chirurgia magna (Great Surgery)*, based on observation and experience, had a profound influence upon the progress of surgery.

The Renaissance in the 14th, 15th, and 16th centuries was much more than just a reviving of interest in Greek and Roman culture. It was rather a change of outlook, an eagerness for discovery, a desire to escape from the limitations of tradition and to explore new fields of thought and action. In medicine, it was perhaps natural that anatomy and physiology, the knowledge of the human body and its workings, should be the first aspects of medical learning to receive attention from those who realized the need for reform.

It was in 1543 that Andreas Vesalius, a young Belgian professor of anatomy at the University of Padua, wrote a text giving groundbreaking evidence based on his own dissections that corrected many of Galen's errors. By his scientific observations and methods, Vesalius showed that Galen could no longer be regarded as the final authority. His work at Padua was continued by Gabriel Fallopius and, later, by Hieronymus Fabricius ab Aquapendente. It was Fabricius' work on the valves in the veins that suggested to his pupil William Harvey his revolutionary theory of the circulation of the blood, one of the great medical discoveries.

Surgery profited from the new outlook in anatomy, and the great reformer Ambroise Paré dominated the field in the 16th century. Paré was surgeon to four kings of France, and he has deservedly been called the father of modern surgery. In his autobiography, written after he had retired from 30 years of service as an army surgeon, Paré described how he had abolished the painful practice of cautery to stop bleeding and used ligatures and dressings instead. His favourite expression, "I dressed him; God healed him," is characteristic of this humane and careful doctor.

In Britain during this period surgery, which was performed by barber-surgeons, was becoming regulated and organized under royal charters. Companies were thus formed that eventually became the royal colleges of surgeons in Scotland and England. Physicians and surgeons united in a joint organization in Glasgow, and a college of physicians was founded in London.

The 16th-century medical scene was enlivened by the enigmatic physician and alchemist who called himself Paracelsus. Born in Switzerland, he traveled extensively throughout Europe, gaining medical skills and practicing and teaching as he went. In the tradition of Hippocrates, Paracelsus stressed the power of nature to heal. But unlike Hippocrates he believed also in the power of supernatural forces, and he violently attacked the medical treatments of his day. Eager for reform, he allowed his intolerance to outweigh his discretion, as when he prefaced his lectures at Basel by publicly burning the works of Avicenna and Galen. The authorities and medical men were understandably outraged. Widely famous in his time, Paracelsus remains a controversial figure to this day. Despite his turbulent career, however, he did attempt to bring a more rational approach to diagnosis and treatment, and he introduced the use of chemical drugs in place of herbal remedies.

A contemporary of Paracelsus, Girolamo Fracastoro of Italy was a scholar cast from a very different mold. His account of the disease syphilis, entitled *Syphilis sive morbus Gallicus* (1530; *Syphilis or the French Disease*), was written in verse. Although Fracastoro called syphilis the French disease, others called it the Neapolitan disease, for it was said to have been brought to Naples from America by the sailors of Christopher Columbus. Its origin is still questioned, however. Fracastoro was interested in epidemic infection, and he offered the first scientific explanation of disease transmission. In his great work, *De contagione et contagiosis morbis* (1546), he theorized that the seeds of certain diseases are imperceptible particles transmitted by air or by contact.

ANDREAS VESALIUS
(b. Dec. 1514, Brussels [now in Belgium]—d. June 1564, island of Zacynthus, Republic of Venice [now in Greece])

Renaissance physician Andreas Vesalius revolutionized the study of biology and the practice of medicine by his careful description of the anatomy of the human body. Basing his observations on dissections he made himself, he wrote and illustrated the first comprehensive textbook of anatomy.

Vesalius, a native of the duchy of Brabant (the southern portion of which is now in Belgium), was from a family of physicians and pharmacists. He attended the Catholic University of Leuven (Louvain) in 1529–33, and from 1533 to 1536 he studied at the medical school of the University of Paris, where he learned to dissect animals. He also had the opportunity to dissect human cadavers, and he devoted much of his time to a study of human bones, at that time easily available in the Paris cemeteries.

In 1536 Vesalius returned to Brabant to spend another year at the Catholic University of Leuven, where the influence of Arab medicine was still dominant. Following the prevailing custom, he prepared, in 1537, a paraphrase of the work of the 10th-century Arab physician, al-Rāzī, probably in fulfillment of the requirements for the bachelor of medicine degree. He then went to the University of Padua, a progressive university with a strong tradition of anatomical dissection. On receiving the M.D. degree the same year, he was appointed a lecturer in surgery with the responsibility of giving anatomical demonstrations. Since he knew that a thorough knowledge of human anatomy was essential to surgery, he devoted much of his time to dissections of cadavers and insisted on doing them himself, instead of relying on untrained assistants.

In January 1540, breaking with the tradition of relying on Galen, Vesalius openly demonstrated his own method—doing dissections himself, learning anatomy from cadavers, and critically evaluating ancient texts. He did so while visiting the University of Bologna. Such methods soon convinced him that Galenic anatomy had not been based on the dissection of the human body, which had been strictly forbidden by the Roman religion. Galenic anatomy, he maintained, was an application to the human form of conclusions drawn from the dissections of animals, mostly dogs, monkeys, or pigs. It was this conclusion that he had the audacity to declare in his teaching as he hurriedly prepared his complete textbook of human anatomy for publication. Early in 1542 he traveled to Venice to supervise the preparation of drawings to illustrate his text, probably in the studio of the great Renaissance artist Titian. The drawings of his dissections were engraved on wood blocks, which he took, together with his manuscript, to Basel, Switz., where his major work *De humani corporis fabrica libri septem* (*The Seven Books on the Structure of the Human Body*) commonly known as the *Fabrica*, was printed in 1543.

In this epochal work, Vesalius deployed all his scientific, humanistic, and aesthetic gifts. The *Fabrica* was a more extensive and accurate description of the human body than any put forward by his predecessors. It gave anatomy a new language, and, in the elegance of its printing and organization, a perfection hitherto unknown.

HIERONYMUS FABRICIUS AB AQUAPENDENTE
(b. May 20, 1537, Acquapendente, Italy—d. May 21, 1619, Padua)

Italian surgeon Hieronymus Fabricius ab Aquapendente was an outstanding Renaissance anatomist who helped found modern embryology.

He spent most of his life at the University of Padua, where he studied under the eminent anatomist Gabriel Fallopius. As Fallopius' successor to the chair of surgery and anatomy (1562–1613), Fabricius built a reputation that attracted students from all of Europe. The English anatomist William Harvey was his pupil. In *De Venarum Ostiolis* (1603; *On the*

Valves of the Veins), Fabricius gave the first clear description of the semilunar valves of the veins, which later provided Harvey with a crucial point in his famous argument for circulation of the blood.

Fabricius' *De Formato Foetu* (1600; *On the Formation of the Fetus*), summarizing his investigations of the fetal development of many animals, including humans, contained the first detailed description of the placenta and opened the field of comparative embryology. He also gave the first full account of the larynx as a vocal organ and was first to demonstrate that the pupil of the eye changes its size.

THE ENLIGHTENMENT

In the 17th century the natural sciences moved forward on a broad front. There were attempts to grapple with the nature of science, as expressed in the works of thinkers like Francis Bacon, René Descartes, and Isaac Newton. New knowledge of chemistry superseded the theory that all things are made up of earth, air, fire, and water, and the old Aristotelian ideas began to be discarded. The supreme 17th-century achievement in medicine was William Harvey's explanation of the circulation of blood.

HARVEY AND THE EXPERIMENTAL METHOD

Born in Folkestone, Eng., William Harvey studied at Cambridge University and then spent several years at Padua, where he came under the influence of Fabricius.

He established a successful medical practice in London and by precise observation and scrupulous reasoning developed his theory of circulation. In 1628 he published his classic book *Exercitatio Anatomica de Motu Cordis et Sanguinis in Animalibus* (*Anatomical Exercise on the Motion of the Heart and Blood in Animals*), often called *De Motu Cordis*.

That the book aroused controversy is not surprising. There were still many who adhered to the teaching of Galen that the blood follows an ebb and flow movement in the blood vessels. Harvey's work was the result of many careful experiments, but few of his critics took the trouble to repeat the experiments, simply arguing in favour of the older view. His second great book, *Exercitationes de generatione animalium* (*Exercises on the Generation of Animals*), published in 1651, laid the foundation of modern embryology.

Harvey's discovery of the circulation of the blood was a landmark of medical progress. The new experimental method by which the results were secured was as noteworthy as the work itself. Following the method described by the philosopher Francis Bacon, he drew the truth from experience and not from authority.

There was one gap in Harvey's argument: he was obliged to assume the existence of the capillary vessels that conveyed the blood from the arteries to the veins. This link in the chain of evidence was supplied by Marcello Malpighi of Bologna (who was born in 1628, the year of publication of *De Motu Cordis*). With a primitive microscope

Malpighi saw a network of tiny blood vessels in the lung of a frog. Harvey also failed to show why the blood circulated. After Robert Boyle had shown that air is essential to animal life, it was Richard Lower who traced the interaction between air and the blood. Eventually the importance of oxygen, which was confused for a time by some as phlogiston, was revealed, although it was not until the late 18th century that the great chemist Antoine-Laurent Lavoisier discovered the essential nature of oxygen and clarified its relation to respiration.

Although the compound microscope had been invented slightly earlier, probably in Holland, its development, like that of the telescope, was the work of Galileo. He was the first to insist upon the value of measurement in science and in medicine, thus replacing theory and guesswork with accuracy. The great Dutch microscopist Antonie van Leeuwenhoek devoted his long life to microscopical studies and was probably the first to see and describe bacteria, reporting his results to the Royal Society of London. In England, Robert Hooke, who was Boyle's assistant and curator to the Royal Society, published his *Micrographia* in 1665, which discussed and illustrated the microscopic structure of a variety of materials.

The Futile Search for an Easy System

Several attempts were made in the 17th century to discover an easy system that would guide the practice of medicine. A substratum of superstition still remained. Richard Wiseman, surgeon to Charles II, affirmed his belief in the "royal touch" as a cure for king's evil, or scrofula, while even the learned English physician Thomas Browne stated that witches really existed. There was, however, a general desire to discard the past and adopt new ideas.

The view of the French philosopher René Descartes that the human body is a machine and that it functions mechanically had its repercussions in medical thought. One group adopting this explanation called themselves the iatrophysicists. Another school, preferring to view life as a series of chemical processes, were called iatrochemists. Santorio Santorio, working at Padua, was an early exponent of the iatrophysical view and a pioneer investigator of metabolism. He was especially concerned with the measurement of what he called "insensible perspiration," described in his book *De statica medicina* (1614; *On Medical Measurement*). Another Italian, who developed the idea still further, was Giovanni Alfonso Borelli, a professor of mathematics at Pisa University, who gave his attention to the mechanics and statics of the body and to the physical laws that govern its movements.

The iatrochemical school was founded at Brussels by Jan Baptist van Helmont, whose writings are tinged with the mysticism of the alchemist. A more logical and intelligible view of iatrochemistry was advanced by Franciscus Sylvius, at Leiden, and in England a leading exponent of the same school was

Thomas Willis, who is better known for his description of the brain in his *Cerebri anatome nervorumque descriptio et usus* (*Anatomy of the Brain and Descriptions and Functions of the Nerves*), published in 1664 and illustrated by Christopher Wren.

It soon became apparent that no easy road to medical knowledge and practice was to be found along these channels and that the best method was the age-old system of straightforward clinical observation initiated by Hippocrates. The need for a return to these views was strongly urged by Thomas Sydenham, well named "the English Hippocrates." Sydenham was not a voluminous writer and, indeed, had little patience with book learning in medicine. Nevertheless he gave excellent descriptions of the phenomena of disease. His greatest service, much needed at the time, was to divert physicians' minds from speculation and lead them back to the bedside, where the true art of medicine could be studied.

MARCELLO MALPIGHI
(b. March 10, 1628, Crevalcore, near Bologna, Papal States [Italy]—d. Nov. 30, 1694, Rome)

Italian physician and biologist Marcello Malpighi developed experimental methods to study living things and thereby founded the science of microscopic anatomy. After Malpighi's researches, microscopic anatomy became a prerequisite for advances in the fields of physiology, embryology, and practical medicine.

Little is known of Malpighi's childhood and youth except that his father had him engage in "grammatical studies" at an early age and that he entered the University of Bologna in 1646. Both parents died when he was 21, but he was able, nevertheless, to continue his studies. Despite opposition from the university authorities because he was non-Bolognese by birth, in 1653 he was granted doctorates in both medicine and philosophy and appointed as a teacher, whereupon he immediately dedicated himself to further study in anatomy and medicine.

In 1656, Ferdinand II of Tuscany invited him to the professorship of theoretical medicine at the University of Pisa. There Malpighi began his lifelong friendship with Giovanni Borelli, mathematician and naturalist, who was a prominent supporter of the Accademia del Cimento, one of the first scientific societies. Malpighi questioned the prevailing medical teachings at Pisa, tried experiments on colour changes in blood, and attempted to recast anatomical, physiological, and medical problems of the day. Family responsibilities and poor health prompted Malpighi's return in 1659 to the University of Bologna, where he continued to teach and do research with his microscopes. In 1661 he identified and described the pulmonary and capillary network connecting small arteries with small veins, one of the major discoveries in the history of science. Malpighi's views evoked increasing controversy and dissent, mainly from envy, jealousy, and lack of understanding on the part of his colleagues.

Hindered by the hostile environment of Bologna, Malpighi accepted (November 1662) a professorship in medicine at the University of Messina in Sicily, on the recommendation there of Borelli, who was investigating the effects of physical forces on animal functions. Malpighi was also welcomed by Visconte Giacomo Ruffo Francavilla, a patron of science and a former student, whose hospitality encouraged him in furthering his career. Malpighi pursued his microscopic studies while teaching and practicing medicine. He identified the taste buds and regarded them as terminations of nerves, described the minute structure of the brain, optic nerve, and fat reservoirs, and in 1666 was the first to see the red blood cells and to attribute the colour of blood to them. Again, his research and teaching aroused envy and controversy among his colleagues.

After four years at Messina, Malpighi returned in January 1667 to Bologna, where, during his medical practice, he studied the microscopic subdivisions of specific living organs, such as the liver, brain, spleen, and kidneys, and of bone and the deeper layers of the skin that now bear his name. Impressed by the minute structures he observed under the microscope, he concluded that most living materials are glandular in organization, that even the largest organs are composed of minute glands, and that these glands exist solely for the separation or for the mixture of juices.

Malpighi's work at Messina attracted the attention of the Royal Society in London, whose secretary, Henry Oldenburg, extended him an invitation in 1668 to correspond with him. Malpighi's work was thereafter published periodically in the form of letters in the *Philosophical Transactions* of the Royal Society. In 1669 Malpighi was named an honorary member, the first such recognition given to an Italian. From then on, all his works were published in London.

While at Bologna Malpighi conducted many studies of insect larvae—establishing, in so doing, the basis for their future study—the most important of which was his investigation in 1669 of the structure and development of the silkworm. In his historic work in 1673 on the embryology of the chick, in which he discovered the aortic arches, neural folds, and somites, he generally followed William Harvey's views on development, though Malpighi probably concluded that the embryo is preformed in the egg after fertilization. He also made extensive comparative studies in 1675–79 of the microscopic anatomy of several different plants and saw an analogy between plant and animal organization.

Malpighi may be regarded as the first histologist. For almost 40 years he used the microscope to describe the major types of plant and animal structures and in so doing marked out for future generations of biologists major areas of research in botany, embryology, human anatomy, and pathology. Just as Galileo had applied the new technical achievement of the optical lens to vistas beyond Earth, Malpighi extended its use to the intricate organization of living things, hitherto unimagined, below the level of unaided sight. Moreover, his lifework brought into question the prevailing concepts of body function. When, for example, he found that the blood passed through the capillaries, it meant that Harvey was right, that blood was not transformed into flesh in the periphery, as the ancients thought. He was vigorously denounced by his enemies, who failed to see how his many discoveries, such as the renal glomeruli, urinary tubules, dermal papillae, taste buds, and the glandular components of the liver, could possibly improve medical practice. The conflict between ancient ideas and modern discoveries continued throughout the 17th century. Although Malpighi could not say what new remedies might come from his discoveries, he was convinced that microscopic anatomy, by showing the minute construction of living things, called into question the value of old medicine. He provided the anatomical basis for the eventual understanding of human physiological exchanges.

SANTORIO SANTORIO
(b. March 29, 1561, Capodistria [now Koper, Slovenia]—d. Feb. 22, 1636, Venice [Italy])

Italian physician Santorio Santorio (Latin: Sanctorius, or Santorius) was the first to employ instruments of precision in the practice of medicine. He also introduced quantitative experimental procedure into medical research through his studies of basal metabolism.

Santorio was a graduate of the University of Padua (M.D., 1582), where he later became professor of medical theory (1611–24). About 1587 he was apparently summoned to attend as physician on a Croatian nobleman. From 1587 to 1599 Santorio seems to have spent much time among the southern Slavs, though he maintained a frequent correspondence with his Paduan colleagues, the astronomer Galileo Galilei and the surgeon and anatomist Hieronymus Fabricius ab Aquapendente. Santorio was an early exponent of the iatrophysical school of medicine, which attempted to explain the workings of the animal body on purely mechanical grounds, and he adapted several of Galileo's inventions to medical practice, resulting in his development of a clinical thermometer (1612) and a pulse clock (1602).

Endeavouring to test the Greek physician Galen's assertion that respiration also occurs through the skin as "insensible perspiration," Santorio constructed a large scale on which he frequently ate, worked, and slept, so that he might study the fluctuations of his body weight in relation to his solid and liquid excretions. After 30 years of continuous experimentation, he found that the sum total of visible excreta was less than the amount of substance ingested. His *De Statica Medicina* (1614; *On Medical Measurement*) was the first systematic study of basal metabolism.

MEDICINE IN THE 18TH CENTURY

Even in the 18th century the search for a simple way of healing the sick continued. In Edinburgh the writer and lecturer John Brown expounded his view that there were only two diseases, sthenic (strong) and asthenic (weak), and two treatments, stimulant and sedative; his chief remedies were alcohol and opium. Lively and heated debates took place between his followers, the Brunonians, and the more orthodox Cullenians (followers of William Cullen, a professor of medicine at Glasgow), and the controversy spread to the medical centres of Europe.

At the opposite end of the scale, at least in regard to dosage, was Samuel Hahnemann of Leipzig, the originator of homeopathy, a system of treatment involving the administration of minute doses of drugs whose effects resemble the effects of the disease being treated. His ideas had a salutary effect upon medical thought at a time when prescriptions were lengthy and doses were large, and his system has had many followers.

By the 18th century the medical school at Leiden had grown to rival that of Padua, and many students were attracted there from abroad. Among them was John Monro, an army surgeon, who resolved that his native city of Edinburgh should have a similar medical school. He specially educated his son Alexander with a view to having him appointed professor of anatomy, and the bold plan was successful. Alexander Monro studied at Leiden under Hermann Boerhaave, the central figure of European medicine and the greatest clinical teacher of his time. Subsequently, three generations of Alexander Monros taught anatomy at Edinburgh University over a continuous period of 126 years. Medical education was increasingly incorporated into the universities of Europe, and Edinburgh became the leading academic centre for medicine in Britain.

In 18th-century London, Scottish doctors were the leaders in surgery and obstetrics. The noted teacher John Hunter conducted extensive researches in comparative anatomy and physiology, founded surgical pathology, and raised surgery to the level of a respectable branch of science. His brother William Hunter, an eminent teacher of anatomy, became famous as an obstetrician. Male doctors were now attending women in childbirth, and the leading obstetrician in London was William Smellie. His well-known *Treatise on the Theory and Practice of Midwifery*, published in three volumes in 1752–64, contained the first systematic discussion on the safe use of obstetrical forceps, which have since saved countless lives. Smellie placed midwifery on a sound scientific footing and helped to establish obstetrics as a recognized medical discipline.

The science of modern pathology also had its beginnings in this century. Giovanni Battista Morgagni of Padua in 1761 published his massive work *De sedibus et causis morborum (The Seats and Causes of Diseases Investigated by*

Anatomy), a description of the appearances found by postmortem examination of almost 700 cases, in which he attempted to correlate the findings after death with the clinical picture in life.

On the basis of work begun in the 18th century, René-Théophile-Hyacinthe Laënnec, a native of Brittany, who practiced medicine in Paris, invented a simple stethoscope designed to listen to chest sounds. Meanwhile a Viennese physician, Leopold Auenbrugger, discovered another method of investigating diseases of the chest, that of percussion. The son of an innkeeper, he is said to have conceived the idea of tapping with the fingers when he recalled that he had used this method to gauge the level of the fluid contents of his father's casks.

One highly significant medical advance, late in the century, was vaccination. Smallpox, disfiguring and often fatal, was widely prevalent. Inoculation, which had been practiced in the East, was popularized in England in 1721–22 by Lady Mary Wortley Montagu, who is best known for her letters. She observed the practice in Turkey, where it produced a mild form of the disease, thus securing immunity, although not without danger. The next step was taken by Edward Jenner, a country practitioner who had been a pupil of John Hunter. In 1796 Jenner began inoculations with material from cowpox (the bovine form of the disease), and when he later inoculated the same subject with smallpox, the disease did not appear. This procedure—vaccination—has been responsible for eradicating the disease.

Public health and hygiene were receiving more attention during the 18th century. Population statistics began to be kept, and suggestions arose concerning health legislation. Hospitals were established for a variety of purposes. In Paris, Philippe Pinel initiated bold reforms in the care of the mentally ill, releasing them from their chains and discarding the long-held notion that insanity was caused by demon possession.

Conditions improved for sailors and soldiers as well. James Lind, a British naval surgeon from Edinburgh, recommended fresh fruits and citrus juices to prevent scurvy, a remedy discovered by the Dutch in the 16th century. When the British navy adopted Lind's advice—decades later—this deficiency disease was eliminated. In 1752 a Scotsman, John Pringle, published his classic *Observations on the Diseases of the Army*, which contained numerous recommendations for the health and comfort of the troops. Serving with the British forces during the War of the Austrian Succession, he suggested in 1743 that military hospitals on both sides should be regarded as sanctuaries. This plan eventually led to the establishment of the Red Cross organization in 1864.

Two pseudoscientific doctrines relating to medicine emerged from Vienna in the latter part of the century and attained wide notoriety. Mesmerism, a belief in "animal magnetism" sponsored by Franz Anton Mesmer, probably owed any therapeutic value it had to suggestions given while the patient was under hypnosis. Phrenology, propounded by Franz Joseph

MIDWIFERY

Midwifery is the art and practice of attending upon women in childbirth. The profession of midwife must be one of the oldest, being clearly recognized in the earliest books of the Old Testament and an accepted element in the social structure in ancient Greece and Rome. But the old obstetrical learning, meagre as it was, disappeared in the Middle Ages, and the little that survived became adulterated by superstition. Childbirth in those days was associated with an appalling infant mortality and with grave danger to any mother who was unable to deliver herself expeditiously and unaided.

In Europe in the 17th century a slow and hesitant movement for the training of midwives began. In the 18th century, maternity hospitals appeared in the larger cities and became training centres for midwives. It was not until the 19th century that the training and control of midwives' practice were put on a statutory basis. The Netherlands, Scandinavia, Germany, and France all made early progress in this regard. In Great Britain, the first Midwives Act (1902) set up a Central Midwives Board to prescribe the training of student-midwives in hospitals, examine and license candidates, and regulate the practice of all such certified midwives. This was a great advance, for at that time the great majority of births in Great Britain were home births attended by midwives. The Midwives Act resulted in a steady rise in the professional skill of British midwives, most of whom were trained as state registered nurses (S.R.N.) before becoming state certified midwives (S.C.M.).

In the late 19th and early 20th century, advances in obstetrics and gynecology caused a great shift in childbearing from the home to the hospital in most Western nations. In the 1960s, however, a variety of economic and social factors spurred a renewed interest in the concerned, personal care provided by midwives and gave rise, in the United States, to the profession of nurse-midwife. A certified nurse-midwife (C.N.M.) is a registered nurse who has received professional training in midwifery and been certified by the American College of Nurse-Midwives. C.N.M.'s accept only those patients who can be expected to have a normal delivery. They do not perform operative deliveries, and if a delivery does prove difficult, a physician is usually called. C.N.M.'s deliver babies in hospitals, clinics, birthing centres, or, more rarely, at home. They provide prenatal and postnatal care, advise women about their reproductive health before and after pregnancy, and offer family-planning services and counseling.

Lay midwives, by contrast, usually have no professional training in midwifery, are unlicensed, and deliver babies at home. In developed nations, they have traditionally worked in isolated rural areas, but in developing countries they are much more common. Midwives of all sorts deliver about three-fourths of all the infants born throughout the world each year.

Gall, held that the contours of the skull were a guide to an individual's mental faculties and character traits. This theory remained popular throughout the 19th century.

At the same time, sound scientific thinking was making steady progress, and advances in physics, chemistry, and the biological sciences were converging to form a rational scientific basis for every branch of clinical medicine. New knowledge disseminated thoughout Europe and traveled across the sea, where centres of medical excellence were being established in America.

MAJOR FIGURES IN 18TH-CENTURY MEDICINE

The 18th century was a period characterized by substantial growth and expansion in medical and scientific knowledge. This growth was influenced by the work of many physicians, some of whom developed new instruments for diagnosis and treatment and others of whom contributed new theories to the understanding of health and disease. Some of the most notable physicians and medical thinkers of the era included William Cullen, Edward Jenner, René-Théophile-Hyacinthe Laënnec, Benjamin Rush, and Lazzaro Spallanzani.

WILLIAM CULLEN
(b. April 15, 1710, Hamilton, Lanarkshire, Scot.—d. Feb. 5, 1790, Kirknewton, near Edinburgh)

Scottish physician and professor of medicine William Cullen was best known for his innovative teaching methods.

Cullen received his early education at Hamilton Grammar School, in the town where he was born and where his father, a lawyer, was employed by the duke of Hamilton. In 1726 Cullen went to the University of Glasgow, where he became a student of British surgeon John Paisley. In 1729 Cullen was hired to serve as ship's surgeon aboard a merchant vessel sailing from London to the West Indies. Upon his return to London, he took a post as an assistant to a local apothecary. Cullen remained in London until 1732, when he ventured home to Scotland and established his own medical practice near the village of Shotts in Lanarkshire (now North Lanarkshire). In 1734 he attended the new medical school at Edinburgh, returning to his private practice in Hamilton two years later. He spent eight years in private clinical practice, attending without fee those too poor to afford his services. In 1740 he received an M.D. from Glasgow, and several years later he obtained permission to deliver a series of independent lectures on chemistry and medicine, the first to be offered in Great Britain. He was elected to the chair of medicine at Glasgow in 1751. In 1755 Cullen returned to the University of Edinburgh, where he was later appointed to the chair of the institutes (theory) of medicine and eventually became sole professor of medicine, the position he held until shortly before his death. In 1777 Cullen was elected a fellow of the Royal Society of London.

Cullen was considered a progressive thinker for his time. He was the first to demonstrate in public the refrigeration effects of evaporative cooling, a phenomenon he wrote of in "Of the Cold Produced by Evaporating Fluids and of Some Other Means of Producing Cold" (*Essays and Observations, Physical and*

Literary, vol. 2 [1756]). In medicine he taught that life was a function of nervous energy and that muscle was a continuation of nerve. He organized an influential classification of disease (nosology) consisting of four major divisions: pyrexiae, or febrile diseases; neuroses, or nervous diseases; cachexiae, diseases arising from bad bodily habits; and locales, or local diseases. This system, which Cullen described in his work *Synopsis Nosologiae Methodicae* (1769), was based on the observable symptoms that arise from disease and that are utilized for diagnosis.

Cullen was most famous, however, for his innovative teaching methods and forceful, inspiring lectures, which drew medical students to Edinburgh from throughout the English-speaking world. He was one of the first to teach in English rather than in Latin, and he delivered his clinical lectures in the infirmary, lecturing not from a text but from his own notes. His *First Lines of the Practice of Physic* (1777) was widely used as a textbook in Britain and the United States.

Many of Cullen's pupils went on to make important contributions to science and medicine. Among his most well-known students were British chemist and physicist Joseph Black, known for the rediscovery of "fixed air" (carbon dioxide); English physician William Withering, known for his medical discoveries concerning the use of extracts of foxglove (*Digitalis purpurea*); British physician John Brown, who was a propounder of the "excitability" theory of

medicine; and American physician and political leader Benjamin Rush, who was known for his advocacy for the humane treatment of the insane.

EDWARD JENNER
(b. May 17, 1749, Berkeley, Gloucestershire, Eng.—d. Jan. 26, 1823, Berkeley)

English surgeon Edward Jenner is best known as the discoverer of the vaccination for smallpox.

Jenner was a country youth, the son of a clergyman. Because Edward was only five when his father died, he was brought up by an older brother, who was also a clergyman. Edward acquired a love of nature that remained with him all his life. He attended grammar school and at the age of 13 was apprenticed to a nearby surgeon. In the following eight years Jenner acquired a sound knowledge of medical and surgical practice. On completing his apprenticeship at the age of 21, he went to London and became the house pupil of John Hunter, who was on the staff of St. George's Hospital and was one of the most prominent surgeons in London. Even more important, however, he was an anatomist, biologist, and experimentalist of the first rank. Not only did he collect biological specimens, but he also concerned himself with problems of physiology and function.

The firm friendship that grew between the two men lasted until Hunter's death in 1793. From no one else could Jenner have received the stimuli that so confirmed his natural bent—a catholic interest in biological phenomena, disciplined powers of observation, sharpening of critical faculties, and a reliance on experimental investigation. From Hunter, Jenner received the characteristic advice, "Why think [i.e., speculate]—why not try the experiment?"

In addition to his training and experience in biology, Jenner made progress in clinical surgery. After studying in London from 1770 to 1773, he returned to country practice in Berkeley and enjoyed substantial success. He was capable, skillful, and popular. In addition to practicing medicine, he joined two medical groups for the promotion of medical knowledge and wrote occasional medical papers. He played the violin in a musical club, wrote light verse, and, as a naturalist, made many observations, particularly on the nesting habits of the cuckoo and on bird migration. He also collected specimens for Hunter. Many of Hunter's letters to Jenner have been preserved, but Jenner's letters to Hunter have unfortunately been lost. After one disappointment in love in 1778, Jenner married in 1788.

Smallpox was widespread in the 18th century, and occasional outbreaks of special intensity resulted in a very high death rate. The disease, a leading cause of death at the time, respected no social class, and disfigurement was not uncommon in patients who recovered. The only means of combating smallpox was a primitive form of vaccination called variolation—intentionally infecting a healthy person with the "matter" taken

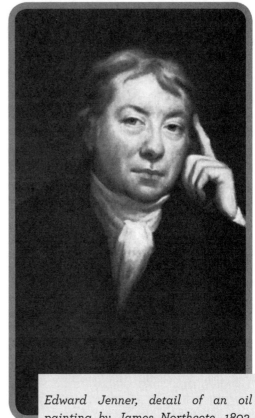

Edward Jenner, detail of an oil painting by James Northcote, 1803. Courtesy of the National Portrait Gallery, London

from a patient sick with a mild attack of the disease. The practice, which originated in China and India, was based on two distinct concepts: first, that one attack of smallpox effectively protected against any subsequent attack and, second, that a person deliberately infected with a mild case of the disease would safely acquire such protection. It was, in present-day terminology, an "elective" infection—i.e., one given to a person in good health. Unfortunately, the transmitted disease did not always remain mild, and mortality sometimes occurred. Furthermore, the inoculated person could disseminate the disease to others and thus act as a focus of infection.

Jenner had been impressed by the fact that a person who had suffered an attack of cowpox—a relatively harmless disease that could be contracted from cattle—could not take the smallpox—i.e., could not become infected whether by accidental or intentional exposure to smallpox. Pondering this phenomenon, Jenner concluded that cowpox not only protected against smallpox but could be transmitted from one person to another as a deliberate mechanism of protection.

The story of the great breakthrough is well known. In May 1796 Jenner found a young dairymaid, Sarah Nelmes, who had fresh cowpox lesions on her hand. On May 14, using matter from Sarah's lesions, he inoculated an eight-year-old boy, James Phipps, who had never had smallpox. Phipps became slightly ill over the course of the next 9 days but was well on the 10th. On July 1 Jenner inoculated the boy again, this time with smallpox matter. No disease developed; protection was complete. In 1798 Jenner, having added further cases, published privately a slender book entitled *An Inquiry into the Causes and Effects of the Variolae Vaccinae.*

The reaction to the publication was not immediately favourable. Jenner went to London seeking volunteers for vaccination but, in a stay of three months, was not successful. In London vaccination became popularized through the activities of others, particularly the surgeon Henry Cline, to whom Jenner had given some of the inoculant, and the doctors George Pearson and William Woodville. Difficulties arose, some of them quite unpleasant. Pearson tried to take credit away from Jenner, and Woodville, a physician in a smallpox hospital, contaminated the cowpox matter with smallpox virus. Vaccination rapidly proved its value, however, and Jenner became intensely active promoting it. The procedure spread rapidly to America and the rest of Europe and soon was carried around the world.

Complications were many. Vaccination seemed simple, but the vast number of persons who practiced it did not necessarily follow the procedure that Jenner had recommended, and deliberate or unconscious innovations often impaired the effectiveness. Pure cowpox vaccine was not always easy to obtain, nor was it easy to preserve or transmit. Furthermore, the biological factors that produce immunity were not yet understood. Much information had to be gathered and a great many mistakes made before a fully effective procedure could be developed, even on an empirical basis.

Despite errors and occasional chicanery, the death rate from smallpox plunged. Jenner received worldwide recognition and many honours, but he made no attempt to enrich himself through his discovery and actually devoted so much time to the cause of vaccination that his private practice and personal affairs suffered severely. Parliament voted him a sum of £10,000 in 1802 and a further sum of £20,000 in 1806. Jenner not only received honours but also aroused opposition and found himself subjected to attacks and calumnies, despite which he continued his activities on behalf of vaccination. His wife, ill with tuberculosis, died in 1815, and Jenner retired from public life.

RENÉ-THÉOPHILE-HYACINTHE LAËNNEC
(b. Feb. 17, 1781, Quimper, Brittany, France—d. Aug. 13, 1826, Kerlouanec)

French physician René-Théophile-Hyacinthe Laënnec invented the stethoscope and perfected the art of auditory examination of the chest cavity.

When Laënnec was five years old, his mother, Michelle Félicité Guesdon, died from tuberculosis, leaving Laënnec and his brother, Michaud, in the incompetent care of their father, Théophile-Marie Laënnec, who worked as a civil servant and had a reputation for reckless spending. In 1793, during the French Revolution, Laënnec went to live with his uncle, Guillaume-François Laënnec, in the port city of Nantes, located in the Pays de la Loire region of western France. Laënnec's uncle was the dean of medicine at the University of Nantes. Although the region was in the midst of counter-revolutionary revolts, the young Laënnec settled into his academic training and, under his uncle's direction, began his medical studies. His first experience working in a hospital setting was at the Hôtel-Dieu of Nantes, where he learned

to apply surgical dressings and to care for patients. In 1800 Laënnec went to Paris and entered the École Pratique, studying anatomy and dissection in the laboratory of surgeon and pathologist Guillaume Dupuytren. Dupuytren was a bright and ambitious academic who became known for his many surgical accomplishments and for his work in alleviating permanent tissue contracture in the palm, a condition later named Dupuytren contracture. While Dupuytren undoubtedly influenced Laënnec's studies, Laënnec also received instruction from other well-known French anatomists and physicians, including Gaspard Laurent Bayle, who studied tuberculosis and cancer; Marie-François-Xavier Bichat, who helped establish histology, the study of tissues; and Jean-Nicolas Corvisart des Marets, who used chest percussion to assess heart function and who served as personal physician to Napoleon I.

Laënnec became known for his studies of peritonitis, amenorrhea, the prostate gland, and tubercle lesions. He graduated in 1804 and continued his research as a faculty member of the Society of the School of Medicine in Paris. He wrote several articles on pathological anatomy and became devoted to Roman Catholicism, which led to his appointment as personal physician to Joseph Cardinal Fesch, half brother of Napoleon and French ambassador to the Vatican in Rome. Laënnec remained Fesch's physician until 1814, when the cardinal was exiled after Napoleon's empire fell. While Laënnec's embrace of

Catholic doctrine was viewed favourably by royalists, many in the medical profession criticized his conservatism, which contradicted the views of many academicians. Nonetheless, Laënnec's restored faith inspired him to find better ways to care for people, especially the poor. From 1812 to 1813, during the Napoleonic Wars, Laënnec took charge of the wards in the Salpêtrière Hospital in Paris, which was reserved for wounded soldiers. After the return of the monarchy, in 1816 Laënnec was appointed as physician at the Necker Hospital in Paris, where he developed the stethoscope.

Laënnec's original stethoscope design consisted of a hollow tube of wood that was 3.5 cm (1.4 inches) in diameter and 25 cm (10 inches) long and was monoaural, transmitting sound to one ear. It could be easily disassembled and reassembled, and it used a special plug to facilitate the transmission of sounds from the patient's heart and lungs. His instrument replaced the practice of immediate auscultation, in which the physician laid his ear on the chest of the patient to listen to chest sounds. The awkwardness that this method created in the case of women patients compelled Laënnec to find a better way to listen to the chest. His wooden monoaural stethoscope was replaced by models using rubber tubing at the end of the 19th century. Other advancements include the development of binaural stethoscopes, capable of transmitting sounds to both ears of the physician.

In 1819 Laënnec published *De l'auscultation médiate* ("On Mediate Auscultation"), the first discourse on a variety of heart and lung sounds heard through the stethoscope. The first English translation of *De l'auscultation médiate* was published in London in 1821. Laënnec's treatise aroused intense interest, and physicians from throughout Europe came to Paris to learn about Laënnec's diagnostic tool. He became an internationally renowned lecturer. In 1822 Laënnec was appointed chair and professor of medicine at the College of France, and the following year he became a full member of the French Academy of Medicine and a professor at the medical clinic of the Charity Hospital in Paris. In 1824 he was made a chevalier of the Legion of Honour. That same year Laënnec married Jacquette Guichard, a widow. They did not have any children, his wife having suffered a miscarriage. Two years later at the age of 45 Laënnec died from cavitating tuberculosis—the same disease that he helped elucidate using his stethoscope. Using his own invention, he could diagnose himself and understand that he was dying.

Because Laënnec's stethoscope enabled heart and lung sounds to be heard without placing an ear on the patient's chest, the stethoscope technique became known as the "mediate" method for auscultation. Throughout Laënnec's medical work and research, his diagnoses were supported with observations and findings from autopsies. In addition to revolutionizing the diagnosis of lung disorders, Laënnec introduced many terms still used today. For example,

Laënnec's cirrhosis, used to describe micronodular cirrhosis (growth of small masses of tissue in the liver that cause degeneration of liver function), and *melanose* (Greek, meaning "black"), which he coined in 1804 to describe melanoma. Laënnec was the first to recognize that melanotic lesions were the result of metastatic melanoma, in which cancer cells from the original tumour site spread to other organs and tissues in the body. He is considered the father of clinical auscultation, and he wrote the first descriptions of pneumonia, bronchiectasis, pleurisy, emphysema, and pneumothorax. His classification of pulmonary conditions is still used today.

BENJAMIN RUSH
(b. Jan. 4, 1746, Byberry, near Philadelphia—d. April 19, 1813, Philadelphia, Pa., U.S.)

American physician and political leader Benjamin Rush was a member of the Continental Congress and a signer of the Declaration of Independence. His encouragement of clinical research and instruction was frequently offset by his insistence upon bloodletting, purging, and other debilitating therapeutic measures.

Rush was born into a pious Presbyterian family. He was sent to a private academy and on to the College of New Jersey at Princeton, from which he was graduated in 1760. After a medical apprenticeship of six years, he sailed for Europe. He took a medical degree at the University of Edinburgh in 1768 and then worked in London hospitals and briefly visited Paris.

Returning home to begin medical practice in 1769, he was appointed professor of chemistry in the College of Philadelphia, and in the following year he published his *Syllabus of a Course of Lectures on Chemistry*, the first American textbook in this field. Despite war and political upheavals, Rush's practice grew to substantial proportions, partly owing to his literary output. The standard checklist of early American medical imprints lists 65 publications under his name, not counting scores of communications to newspapers and magazines. Another source of Rush's professional prestige was the large number of his private apprentices and students from all over the country. He taught some 3,000 students during his tenure as professor of, successively, chemistry, the theory and practice of medicine, and the institutes of medicine and clinical medicine in the College of Philadelphia and the University of Pennsylvania. After 1790 his lectures were among the leading cultural attractions of the city.

As a physician, Rush was a theorist, and a dogmatic one, rather than a scientific pathologist. Striving for a simple, unitary explanation of disease, he conjectured that all diseases are really one—a fever brought on by overstimulation of the blood vessels—and hence subject to a simple remedy—"depletion" by bloodletting and purges. The worse the fever, he believed, the more "heroic" the treatment it called for. In the epidemics of yellow fever that afflicted Philadelphia in the 1790s his cures were more dreaded by some than the disease.

In psychiatry Rush's contributions were more enduring. For many years he laboured among the insane patients at the Pennsylvania Hospital, advocating humane treatment for them on the ground that mental disorders were as subject to healing arts as physical ones. Indeed, he held that insanity often proceeded from physical causes, an idea that was a long step forward from the old notion that lunatics are possessed by devils. His *Medical Inquiries and Observations upon the Diseases of the Mind*, published in 1812, was the first and for many years the only American treatise on psychiatry.

Rush was an early and active American patriot. As a member of the radical provincial conference in June 1776, he drafted a resolution urging independence and was soon elected to the Continental Congress, signing the Declaration of Independence with other members on August 2. For a year he served in the field as surgeon general and physician general of the Middle Department of the Continental Army, but early in 1778 he resigned because he considered the military hospitals mismanaged by his superior, who was supported by General Washington. Rush went on to question Washington's military judgment, a step that he was to regret and one that clouded his reputation until recent times. He resumed the practice and teaching of medicine and in 1797, by appointment of

Pres. John Adams, took on the duties of treasurer of the U.S. Mint. He held this office until his death.

LAZZARO SPALLANZANI
(b. Jan. 12, 1729, Modena, Duchy of Modena—d. 1799, Pavia, Cisalpine Republic)

Italian physiologist Lazzaro Spallanzani made important contributions to the experimental study of bodily functions and animal reproduction. His investigations into the development of microscopic life in nutrient culture solutions paved the way for the research of Louis Pasteur.

Spallanzani was the son of a distinguished lawyer. He attended the Jesuit college at Reggio, where he received a sound education in the classics and philosophy. He was invited to join the order, but, although he was eventually ordained (in 1757), he declined this offer and went to Bologna to study law. Under the influence of his kinswoman Laura Bassi, a professor of mathematics, he became interested in science. In 1754 Spallanzani was appointed professor of logic, metaphysics, and Greek at Reggio College and in 1760 professor of physics at the University of Modena.

Although Spallanzani published in 1760 an article critical of a new translation of the *Iliad*, all of his leisure was being devoted to scientific research. In 1766 he published a monograph on the mechanics of stones that bounce when thrown obliquely across water. His first biological work, published in 1767, was an attack on the biological theory suggested by Georges Buffon and John Turberville Needham, who believed that all living things contain, in addition to inanimate matter, special "vital atoms" that are responsible for all physiological activities. They postulated that, after death, the "vital atoms" escape into the soil and are again taken up by plants. The two men claimed that the small moving objects seen in pond water and in infusions of plant and animal matter are not living organisms but merely "vital atoms" escaping from the organic material. Spallanzani studied various forms of microscopic life and confirmed the view of Antonie van Leeuwenhoek that such forms are living organisms. In a series of experiments he showed that gravy, when boiled, did not produce these forms if placed in phials that were immediately sealed by fusing the glass. As a result of this work, he concluded that the objects in pond water and other preparations were living organisms introduced from the air and that Buffon's views were without foundation.

The range of Spallanzani's experimental interest expanded. The results of his regeneration and transplantation experiments appeared in 1768. He studied regeneration in a wide range of animals including planarians, snails, and amphibians and reached a number of general conclusions: the lower animals have greater regenerative power than the higher; young individuals have a greater capacity for regeneration than the adults

of the same species; and, except in the simplest animals, it is the superficial parts not the internal organs that can regenerate. His transplantation experiments showed great experimental skill and included the successful transplant of the head of one snail onto the body of another. In 1773 he investigated the circulation of the blood through the lungs and other organs and did an important series of experiments on digestion, in which he obtained evidence that digestive juice contains special chemicals that are suited to particular foods.

At the request of his friend Charles Bonnet, Spallanzani investigated the male contribution to generation. Although the spermatozoa had first been seen in the 17th century, their function was not understood until some 30 years after the formulation of the cell theory in 1839. As a result of his earlier investigations into simple animals, Spallanzani supported the prevailing view that the spermatozoa were parasites within the semen. Both Bonnet and Spallanzani accepted the preformation theory. According to their version of this theory, the germs of all living things were created by God in the beginning and were encapsulated within the first female of each species. Thus, the new individual present in each egg was not formed *de novo* but developed as the result of an expansion of parts the delineation of which had been laid down within the germ by God at the creation. It was assumed that the semen provided a stimulus for this expansion, but it was not known if contact was essential nor if all the parts of the semen were required. Using amphibians, Spallanzani showed that actual contact between egg and semen is essential for the development of a new animal and that filtered semen becomes less and less effective as filtration becomes more and more complete. He noted that the residue on the filter paper retained all its original power if it were immediately added to the water containing the eggs. Spallanzani concluded that it was the solid parts of the secretion, proteinaceous and fatty substances that form the bulk of the semen, that were essential, and he continued to regard the spermatozoa as inessential parasites. Despite this error, Spallanzani performed some of the first successful artificial insemination experiments on lower animals and on a dog.

Toward the end of his life he conducted further research on microscopic animals and plants that he had started early in his career. He also began studies on the electric charge of the torpedo fish and sense organs in bats. In his last set of experiments, published posthumously, he attempted to show that the conversion of oxygen to carbon dioxide must occur in tissues, not in the lungs (as Antoine-Laurent Lavoisier had suggested in 1787).

CHAPTER 3

THE RISE OF SCIENTIFIC MEDICINE IN THE 19TH CENTURY

The portrayal of the history of medicine becomes more difficult in the 19th century. Discoveries multiply, and the number of eminent doctors is so great that the history is apt to become a series of biographies. Nevertheless, it is possible to discern the leading trends in modern medical thought. Major 19th-century advances in medicine included the solidification of physiology as a scientific discipline, the verification of germ theory (the theory that certain diseases are caused by the invasion of the body by microorganisms), and the application of antisepsis and anesthesia in surgery.

EMERGENCE OF PHYSIOLOGY

The word *physiology*—now used to denote the study of the functioning of living organisms, animal or plant, and of the functioning of their constituent tissues or cells—was first used by the Greeks around 600 BCE to describe a philosophical inquiry into the nature of things. The use of the term with specific reference to vital activities of healthy humans, which began in the 16th century, also is applicable to many current aspects of physiology. In the 19th century, curiosity, medical necessity, and economic interest stimulated research concerning the physiology of all living organisms. Discoveries of unity of structure and functions common to all living things resulted in the development of the concept of general physiology, in which general principles and concepts applicable to all living things are sought. Since the mid-19th century, therefore, the word *physiology* has implied the utilization of experimental methods, as well as techniques and concepts of the physical sciences, to investigate causes and mechanisms of the activities of all living things.

The philosophical natural history that comprised the physiology of the Greeks has little in common with modern physiology. Many ideas important in the development of physiology, however, were formulated in the books of the Hippocratic school of medicine (before 350 BCE), especially the humoral theory of disease in the treatise *De natura hominis* ("On the Nature of Man"). Other contributions were made by Aristotle (*Lykaion*, about 325 BCE) and Galen of Pergamum (*c.* 130 CE –*c.* 200 CE). Significant in the history of physiology was the teleology of Aristotle, who assumed that every part of the body is formed for a purpose and that function, therefore, can be deduced from structure. The work of Aristotle was the basis for Galen's *De usu partium* ("On the Use of Parts") and a source for many early misconceptions in physiology. The tidal concept of blood flow, the humoral theory of disease, and Aristotle's teleology, for example, led Galen into a basic misunderstanding of the movements of blood that was not corrected until William Harvey's work on blood circulation in the 17th century.

The publication in 1628 of Harvey's *De Motu Cordis* usually is identified as the beginning of modern experimental physiology. Harvey's study, however, was based only on anatomical experiments. Despite increased knowledge in physics and chemistry during the 17th century, physiology remained closely tied to anatomy and medicine. In 1747 in Berne, Switzerland, Albrecht von Haller, eminent as anatomist, physiologist, and botanist, published the first manual for physiology. Between 1757 and 1766 he published eight volumes entitled *Elementa Physiologiae Corporis Humani* (*Elements of Human Physiology*), all of which were in Latin and characterized his definition of physiology as anatomy in motion. At the end of the 18th century, Antoine Lavoisier wrote about the physiological problems of respiration and the production of heat by animals in a series of memoirs that still serve as a foundation for understanding these subjects.

Physiology as a distinct discipline utilizing chemical, physical, and anatomical methods began to develop in the 19th century. Claude Bernard in France; Johannes Müller, Justus von Liebig, and Carl Ludwig in Germany; and Sir Michael Foster in England may be numbered among the founders of physiology as it now is known. At the beginning of the 19th century, German physiology was under the influence of the romantic school of *Naturphilosophie*. In France, on the other hand, romantic elements were opposed by rational and skeptical viewpoints. Bernard's teacher, François Magendie, the pioneer of experimental physiology, was one of the first men to perform experiments on living animals. Both Müller and Bernard, however, recognized that the results of observations and experiments must be incorporated into a body of scientific knowledge, and that the theories of natural philosophers must be tested by experimentation. Many important ideas in physiology were investigated experimentally by Bernard, who also wrote books on the subject. He recognized cells as functional units of life and developed the concept of blood and body fluids as the internal environment (*milieu intérieur*) in which cells carry out their activities. This concept of physiological regulation of the internal environment occupies an important position in physiology and medicine. Bernard's work had a profound influence on succeeding generations of physiologists in France, Russia, Italy, England, and the United States.

Müller's interests were anatomical and zoological, whereas Bernard's were chemical and medical, but both men sought a broad biological viewpoint in physiology rather than one limited to human functions. Although Müller did not perform many experiments, his textbook *Handbuch der Physiologie des Menschen für Vorlesungen* and his personal influence determined the course of animal biology in Germany during the 19th century.

It has been said that, if Müller provided the enthusiasm and Bernard the ideas for modern physiology, Carl Ludwig provided the methods. During his medical studies at the University of Marburg in Germany, Ludwig applied new ideas and methods of the physical sciences to physiology. In 1847 he invented the kymograph, a cylindrical drum that still is used to record muscular motion, changes in blood pressure, and other physiological phenomena. He also made significant contributions to the physiology of circulation and urine secretion. His textbook of physiology, published in two volumes in 1852 and 1856, was the first to stress physical instead of anatomical orientation in physiology. In 1869 at Leipzig, Ludwig founded the Physiological Institute (*neue physiologische Anstalt*), which served as a model for research institutes in medical schools all over the world. The chemical approach to physiological problems, developed first in France by Lavoisier, was expanded in Germany by Justus von Liebig, whose books on *Organic Chemistry and its Applications to Agriculture and Physiology* (1840) and *Animal Chemistry* (1842) created new areas of study both in medical physiology and agriculture. German schools devoted to the study of physiological chemistry evolved from Liebig's laboratory at Giessen.

The British tradition of physiology is distinct from that of the continental schools. In 1869 Sir Michael Foster became Professor of Practical Physiology at University College in London, where he taught the first laboratory course ever offered as a regular part of instruction in medicine. The pattern Foster established still is followed in medical schools in Great Britain and the United States. In 1870 Foster transferred his activities to

Trinity College at Cambridge, England, and a postgraduate medical school emerged from his physiology laboratory there. Although Foster did not distinguish himself in research, his laboratory produced many of the leading physiologists of the late 19th century in Great Britain and the United States. In 1877 Foster wrote a major book (*Textbook of Physiology*), which passed through seven editions and was translated into German, Italian, and Russian. He also published *Lectures on the History of Physiology* (1901). In 1876, partly in response to increased opposition in England to experimentation with animals, Foster was instrumental in founding the Physiological Society, the first organization of professional physiologists. In 1878, again due largely to Foster's activities, the *Journal of Physiology*, which was the first journal devoted exclusively to the publication of research results in physiology, was initiated.

Foster's teaching methods in physiology and a new evolutionary approach to zoology were transferred to the United States in 1876 by Henry Newell Martin, a professor of biology at Johns Hopkins University in Baltimore, Md. The American tradition drew also on the continental schools. S. Weir Mitchell, who studied under Claude Bernard, and Henry P. Bowditch, who worked with Carl Ludwig, joined Martin to organize the American Physiological Society in 1887, and in 1898 the society sponsored publication of the *American Journal of Physiology*. In 1868 Eduard

Pflüger, professor at the Institute of Physiology at Bonn, founded the *Archiv für die gesammte Physiologie*, which became the most important journal of physiology in Germany.

Physiological chemistry followed a course partly independent of physiology. Müller and Liebig provided a stronger relationship between physical and chemical approaches to physiology in Germany than prevailed elsewhere. Felix Hoppe-Seyler, who founded his *Zeitschrift für physiologische Chemie* in 1877, gave identity to the chemical approach to physiology. The American tradition in physiological chemistry initially followed that in Germany. In England, however, it developed from a Cambridge laboratory founded in 1898 to complement the physical approach started earlier by Foster.

Physiology in the 20th century developed into a mature science. During a century of growth, it became the parent of a number of related disciplines, of which biochemistry, biophysics, general physiology, and molecular biology are the most vigorous examples. Physiology, however, retains an important position among the functional sciences that are closely related to the field of medicine. Although many research areas, especially in mammalian physiology, were fully exploited from a classical-organ and organ-system point of view, comparative studies in physiology continued. In the 21st century, the solution of the major unsolved problems of physiology requires technical and expensive research by teams of specialized investigators. Modern research in physiology is aimed at the integration of the varied activities of cells, tissues, and organs at the level of the intact organism. Both analytical and integrative approaches uncover new problems that also must be solved. In many instances, the solution is of practical value in medicine or helps to improve the understanding of both humans and other animals.

VERIFICATION OF GERM THEORY

Perhaps the overarching medical advance of the 19th century, certainly the most spectacular, was the conclusive demonstration that certain diseases, as well as the infection of surgical wounds, were directly caused by minute living organisms. This discovery changed the whole face of pathology and effected a complete revolution in the practice of surgery.

The idea that disease was caused by entry into the body of imperceptible particles was of ancient date. It had been expressed by the Roman encyclopaedist Varro as early as 100 BCE, by Fracastoro in 1546, by Athanasius Kircher and Pierre Borel about a century later, and by Francesco Redi, who in 1684 wrote his *Osservazioni intorno agli animali viventi che si trovano negli animali viventi* ("Observations on Living Animals Which Are to Be Found Within Other Living Animals"), in which he sought to disprove the idea of spontaneous generation. Everything must have a parent, he wrote; only life produces life. A 19th-century pioneer in this field,

regarded by some as founder of the parasitic theory of infection, was Agostino Bassi of Italy, who showed that a disease of silkworms was caused by a fungus that could be destroyed by chemical agents.

The main credit for establishing the science of bacteriology must be accorded to the French chemist Louis Pasteur. It was Pasteur who, by a brilliant series of experiments, proved that the fermentation of wine and the souring of milk are caused by living microorganisms. His work led to the pasteurization of milk and solved problems of agriculture and industry as well as those of animal and human diseases. He successfully employed inoculations to prevent anthrax in sheep and cattle, chicken cholera in fowl, and finally rabies in humans and dogs. The latter resulted in the widespread establishment of Pasteur institutes.

From Pasteur, Joseph Lister derived the concepts that enabled him to introduce the antiseptic principle into surgery. In 1865 Lister, a professor of surgery at Glasgow University, began placing an antiseptic barrier of carbolic acid between the wound and the germ-containing atmosphere. Infections and deaths fell dramatically, and his pioneering work led to more refined techniques of sterilizing the surgical environment.

Obstetrics had already been robbed of some of its terrors by Alexander Gordon at Aberdeen, Scot., Oliver Wendell Holmes at Boston, and Ignaz Semmelweis at Vienna and Pest (Budapest), who advocated disinfection of the hands and clothing of midwives and medical students who attended con-finements. These measures produced a marked reduction in cases of puerperal fever, the bacterial scourge of women following childbirth.

Another pioneer in bacteriology was the German physician Robert Koch, who showed how bacteria could be cultivated, isolated, and examined in the laboratory. A meticulous investigator, Koch discovered the organisms of tuberculosis, in 1882, and cholera, in 1883. By the end of the century many other disease-producing microorganisms had been identified.

DISCOVERIES IN CLINICAL MEDICINE AND ANESTHESIA

There was perhaps some danger that in the search for bacteria other causes of disease would escape detection. Many physicians, however, were working along different lines in the 19th century. Among them were a group attached to Guy's Hospital, in London: Richard Bright, Thomas Addison, and Sir William Gull. Bright contributed significantly to the knowledge of kidney diseases, including Bright disease, and Addison gave his name to disorders of the adrenal glands and the blood. Gull, a famous clinical teacher, left a legacy of pithy aphorisms that might well rank with those of Hippocrates.

In Dublin Robert Graves and William Stokes introduced new methods in clinical diagnosis and medical training. While in Paris a leading clinician, Pierre-Charles-Alexandre Louis, was attracting many students from America by the excellence of his teaching. By the early 19th century the United States was ready to send back the results of its own researches and breakthroughs. In 1809, in a small Kentucky town, Ephraim McDowell boldly operated on a woman—without anesthesia or antisepsis—and successfully removed a large ovarian tumour. William Beaumont, in treating a shotgun wound of the stomach, was led to make many original observations that were published in 1833 as *Experiments and Observations on the Gastric Juice and the Physiology of Digestion*.

The most famous contribution by the United States to medical progress at this period was undoubtedly the introduction of general anesthesia, a procedure that not only liberated the patient from the fearful pain of surgery but also enabled the surgeon to perform more extensive operations. The discovery was marred by controversy. Crawford Long, Gardner Colton, Horace Wells, and Charles Jackson are all claimants for priority. Some used nitrous oxide gas, and others employed ether, which was less capricious. There is little doubt, however, that it was William Thomas Morton who, on Oct. 16, 1846, at Massachusetts General Hospital, in Boston, first demonstrated before a gathering of physicians the use of ether as a general anesthetic. The news quickly reached Europe, and general anesthesia soon became prevalent in surgery. At Edinburgh, the professor of

CHLOROFORM

Chloroform, also called trichloromethane, is a nonflammable, clear, colourless liquid that is denser than water and has a pleasant etherlike odour. It was first prepared in 1831. The Scottish physician Sir James Simpson of the University of Edinburgh was the first to use it as an anesthetic in 1847. It later captured public notice in 1853 when English physician John Snow administered it to Queen Victoria during the birth of Prince Leopold, her eighth child.

Chloroform has a relatively narrow margin of safety and has been replaced by better inhalation anesthetics. In addition, it is believed to be toxic to the liver and kidneys and may cause liver cancer. Chloroform was once widely used as a solvent, but safety and environmental concerns have reduced this use as well. Nevertheless, chloroform has remained an important industrial chemical.

Chloroform is prepared by the chlorination of methane. The major use of chloroform is in the preparation of chlorodifluoromethane (HCFC-22). HCFC-22 contributes to depletion of the ozone layer, and its production is scheduled to halt by 2020 in the United States. As HCFC-22 production is phased out, chloroform production is expected to decrease significantly.

Chloroform is formed by the reaction of chlorine with organic substances present in water and thus can occur in drinking water that has been chlorinated. The limit set by the U.S. Environmental Protection Agency for chloroform contamination is 80 parts per billion (ppb). A typical municipal water supply contains roughly 50 ppb.

midwifery, James Young Simpson, had been experimenting upon himself and his assistants, inhaling various vapours with the object of discovering an effective anesthetic. In November 1847 chloroform was tried with complete success, and soon it was preferred to ether and became the anesthetic of choice.

ADVANCES AT THE END OF THE 19TH CENTURY

While antisepsis and anesthesia placed surgery on an entirely new footing, similarly important work was carried out in other fields of study, such as parasitology and disease transmission. Patrick

Manson, a British pioneer in tropical medicine, showed in China, in 1877, how insects can carry disease and how the embryos of the *Filaria* worm, which can cause elephantiasis, are transmitted by the mosquito. Manson explained his views to a British army surgeon, Ronald Ross, then working on the problem of malaria, and Ross discovered the malarial parasite in the stomach of the *Anopheles* mosquito in 1897.

In Cuba, Carlos Finlay expressed the view, in 1881, that yellow fever is carried by the *Stegomyia* mosquito. Following his lead, the Americans Walter Reed, William Gorgas, and others were able to conquer the scourge of yellow fever in

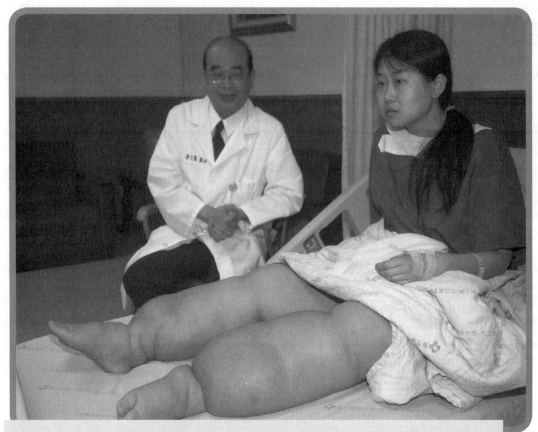

Woman being treated for elephantiasis in Taipei, Taiwan, Republic of China. This rare condition made her legs swell up to triple their normal size. Sam Yeh/AFP/Getty Images

Panama and made possible the completion of the Panama Canal by reducing the death rate there from 176 per 1,000 to 6 per 1,000.

Other victories in preventive medicine ensued, because the maintenance of health was now becoming as important a concern as the cure of disease. The 20th century was to witness the evolution and progress of national health services in a number of countries. In addition, spectacular advances in diagnosis and treatment followed the discovery of X rays by Wilhelm Conrad Röntgen, in 1895, and of radium by Pierre and Marie Curie in 1898. Before the turn of the century, too, the vast new field of psychiatry had been opened up by Sigmund Freud. The tremendous increase in scientific knowledge during the 19th century radically altered and expanded the practice of medicine. Concern for upholding the quality of services led to the establishment of public and professional bodies to govern the standards for medical training and practice.

FILARIAL WORM

Filarial worms are parasitic worms of the family Filariidae (phylum Nematoda) that usually require two hosts, an arthropod (the intermediate host) and a vertebrate (the primary host), to complete the life cycle. The larval phase occurs within the body of a biting insect. The mature (reproductive) phase occurs in the body of an animal bitten by the insect.

The female worm produces large numbers of microscopic, active embryos called microfilariae that pass into the bloodstream of the primary host. The microfilariae may then enter the body of an insect as the insect bites the infected animal. The microfilariae grow into larvae in the insect's muscles and may then be passed to the primary host when the insect bites an animal. The larvae reach adulthood within the vertebrate host, and the cycle repeats. In mammals filarial worms cause a group of infectious disorders including heartworm, elephantiasis, and river blindness. These disorders are known collectively as filariasis. At present, more than 200 million people are infected with filarial parasites.

NOTABLE 19TH-CENTURY PHYSICIANS

The work of prominent 19th-century scientists such as Louis Pasteur and Joseph Lister was supported in large part by the research of individuals in a wide range of medical fields. Collectively, their work was important in establishing and strengthening the scientific basis of medicine and has had an everlasting impact on medical practice. Included among the many important pioneers of 19th-century medicine are Nobelists Jules Bordet and Sir Ronald Ross and English physician and epidemiologist John Snow.

WILLIAM BEAUMONT
(b. Nov. 21, 1785, Lebanon, Conn., U.S.—d. April 25, 1853, St. Louis, Mo.)

American army surgeon William Beaumont was the first person to observe and study human digestion as it occurs in the stomach.

On June 6, 1822, while serving at Fort Mackinac (now in Michigan), Beaumont was summoned to Michilimackinac to treat Alexis St. Martin, a 19-year-old French-Canadian trapper, who had been wounded at close range by a shotgun blast. The shot had removed a portion of the abdominal wall and left a perforation in the anterior wall of the stomach. During the year it took for the wound to heal, the aperture in the abdominal wall never sealed but was held closed by the inversion of tissue surrounding it. As a result, a gastric fistula, or passage, remained. When it was depressed with the finger, Beaumont could view the activities occurring within St. Martin's stomach.

Three years after the near-fatal accident Beaumont began physiological studies of St. Martin's stomach. He believed that the process of digestion was essentially the work of chemicals in the stomach. Determined to prove this hypothesis, he collected samples of gastric juice and sent them for analysis to several chemists, who established the presence of free hydrochloric acid in the juice. Beaumont also reported on the effects of different foods on the stomach, finding that vegetables were less digestible than other foods, that milk coagulated prior to the onset of digestion, and that cold gastric juice had no effect upon food. In 1833 he published *Experiments and Observations on the Gastric Juice and the Physiology of Digestion*. Beaumont's experiments threw new light upon the nature of gastric juice and the digestive process in general, and established alcohol as a cause of gastritis (inflammation of the stomach's mucous membrane).

CLAUDE BERNARD
(b. July 12, 1813, Saint-Julien, France—d. Feb. 10, 1878, Paris)

French physiologist Claude Bernard was known chiefly for his discoveries concerning the role of the pancreas in digestion, the glycogenic function of the liver, and the regulation of the blood supply by the vasomotor nerves. On a broader stage, Bernard played a role in establishing the principles of experimentation in the life sciences, advancing beyond the vitalism and indeterminism of earlier physiologists to become one of the founders of experimental medicine. His most seminal contribution was his concept of the internal environment of the organism,

which led to the present understanding of homeostasis—i.e., the self-regulation of vital processes.

In the winter of 1834-35 Bernard enrolled in the Faculty of Medicine in Paris and, in due course, was admitted as an extern in the hospitals. Outwardly reserved and even shy at that time, he had an inner strength that was to overcome poverty and discouragements. Of 29 students passing the examination for the internship, Bernard ranked 26th. Serving in Paris hospitals were the celebrated doctors Pierre Rayer and François Magendie, and Bernard studied under the latter at both the Hôtel-Dieu and the Collège de France. Magendie noticed Bernard's skillful dissections and took him on as a research assistant.

Bernard became involved in Magendie's research on spinal nerves. His first publication dealt with the chorda tympani (a branch of the facial nerve), while his medical dissertation was devoted to the function of the gastric juice in nutrition (1843). These maiden publications were prophetic, for much of his later research concerned neurology and metabolism. Failing in the examination that would have qualified him to teach in the medical school, he collaborated with others in research on digestion and on the exotic poison curare, thus treading two paths that would lead him to fame. He was rather old at the age of 31 to be content with a research assistantship, however, and resigned the position late in 1844. Left in financial straits, he turned his thoughts again toward medical practice.

In 1847 Bernard became Magendie's deputy at the Collège de France. This period was marked by a veritable explosion of discoveries, beginning in 1846, when Bernard solved the mystery of the carnivorous rabbits. Puzzled one day by the chance observation that some rabbits were passing clear—not cloudy—urine, just like meat-eating animals, he inferred that they had not been fed and were subsisting on their own tissues. He confirmed his hypothesis by feeding meat to the famished animals. An autopsy of the rabbits yielded an important discovery concerning the role of the pancreas in digestion: the secretions of the pancreas broke down fat molecules into fatty acids and glycerin. Bernard then showed that the principal processes of digestion take place in the small intestine, not in the stomach as was previously believed.

His work on the pancreas led to research on the liver, culminating in his second great discovery, the glycogenic function of the liver. In 1856 Bernard discovered glycogen, a white starchy substance found in the liver. He found that this complex substance was built up by the body from sugar and served as a storage reserve of carbohydrates that could be broken down to sugars as needed, thereby keeping the sugar content of the blood at a constant level. Bernard's discovery showed that the digestive system not only breaks down complex molecules into simple ones but also does the opposite, building up complex molecules from simpler ones. Simultaneously, he was nearing his third great achievement—explanation of the regulation of the blood supply by the vasomotor nerves. He discovered in this regard that the vasomotor nerves control the dilation and constriction of blood vessels in response to temperature changes in the environment. For example, in cold weather the blood vessels of the skin constrict in order to conserve heat, while in hot weather they expand to dissipate excess heat. This control mechanism, like the glycogenic functions of the liver, illustrates how the body maintains a stable internal environment in the midst of changing external conditions— a fundamental phenomenon known as homeostasis.

Bernard also conducted important studies on the effects of such poisons as carbon monoxide and curare on the body. He showed that carbon monoxide could substitute for oxygen and combine with hemoglobin, thereby causing oxygen starvation. His experiments with curare showed how this dread poison causes paralysis and death by attacking the motor nerves, while having no effect on the sensory nerves. He demonstrated that, because of this selectivity, curare could be used as an experimental tool in differentiating neuromuscular from primary muscular mechanisms.

In 1854 a chair of general physiology was created for him in the Sorbonne, and he was elected to the Academy of Sciences. When Magendie died in 1855, Bernard succeeded him as full professor at the Collège de France. No laboratory had been provided for Bernard at the Sorbonne, but the French emperor

Napoleon III, after an interview with him in 1864, remedied the deficiency, at the same time building a laboratory at the Museum of Natural History of the Jardin des Plantes. In 1868 Bernard left the Sorbonne to accept a newly established professorship in general physiology at this museum. Bernard suffered apparently from chronic enteritis, with symptoms affecting the pancreas and the liver. By way of compensation, the enforced leisure left him time for reflection, out of which would come his masterpiece, *Introduction à la médecine expérimentale* (1865; *An Introduction to the Study of Experimental Medicine*).

Bernard's aim in the *Introduction* was to demonstrate that medicine, in order to progress, must be founded on experimental physiology. The other points in his argument are that (1) the physical and chemical sciences provide the foundation for physiology, although it is not reducible to them; (2) the notion of "vital force" does not explain life; (3) vivisection is indispensable for physiological research; and (4) biology depends on recognizing that the processes of life are mechanistically determined by physico-chemical forces. Still germane for modern science is his presentation of the concept of the *milieu intérieur*, or "internal environment," of the body. The book brought new honours to Bernard, notably election to the French Academy in 1868.

The most renowned of the students trained by Bernard were Albert Dastre, Paul Bert, and Arsène d'Arsonval. Bert succeeded Bernard in the Sorbonne when the latter transferred to the Museum of Natural History in 1868. Bernard's own experiments were taking new directions. The phenomena common to animals and plants formed the subject of lectures published posthumously. He also began research on fermentation. His findings were published after his death by Berthelot and, because they conflicted with Pasteur's views, cast a cloud over the microbe hunter's memory of his late colleague.

JULES BORDET
(b. June 13, 1870, Soignies, Belg.—d. April 6, 1961, Brussels)

Belgian physician, bacteriologist, and immunologist Jules Bordet received the Nobel Prize for Physiology or Medicine in 1919 for his discovery of factors in blood serum that destroy bacteria. This work was vital to the diagnosis and treatment of many dangerous contagious diseases.

Bordet's research on the destruction of bacteria and red corpuscles in blood serum, conducted at the Pasteur Institute, Paris (1894–1901), contributed significantly to the foundation of serology, the study of immune reactions in body fluids. In 1895 he found that two components of blood serum are responsible for the rupture of bacterial cell walls (bacteriolysis): one is a heat-stable antibody found only in animals already immune to the bacterium; the other is a heat-sensitive substance found in all animals and was named alexin (it is now called complement). Three years later Bordet discovered that red blood cells from one animal species that are injected into another species are destroyed through a process (hemolysis) analogous to bacteriolysis.

In Brussels, where Bordet founded and directed (1901–40) what is now the Pasteur Institute of Brussels, he continued his immunity research with Octave Gengou, his brother-in-law. Their work led to the development of the complement-fixation test, a diagnostic technique that was used to detect the presence of infectious agents in the blood, including those that cause typhoid, tuberculosis, and, most notably, syphilis (the Wassermann test). After discovering (with Gengou in 1906) the bacterium, now known as *Bordetella pertussis*, that is responsible for whooping cough, Bordet became professor of bacteriology at the Free University of Brussels (1907–35).

GARDNER QUINCY COLTON
(b. Feb. 7, 1814, Georgia, Vt., U.S.—d. Aug. 9, 1898, Rotterdam, Neth.)

American anesthetist and inventor Gardner Quincy Colton was among the first to utilize the anesthetic properties

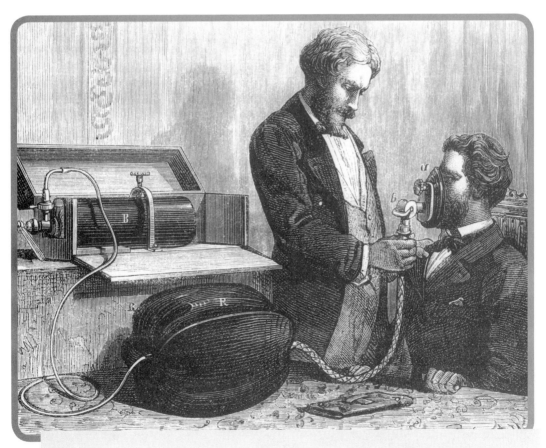

This 1874 plate shows a patient inhaling laughing gas. SSPL via Getty Images

of nitrous oxide in medical practice. After a dentist suggested the use of the gas as an anesthetic, Colton safely used it in extracting thousands of teeth.

As he was studying medicine in New York (without taking a degree), Colton learned that the inhalation of nitrous oxide, or laughing gas, produced exhilaration. After a public demonstration of its effects in New York City proved to be a financial success, he began a lecture tour of other cities. On Dec. 10, 1844, at a Hartford, Conn., demonstration, Horace Wells, a dentist, asked Colton to extract one of his teeth while he was under the effects of the gas. Wells began using the gas in his dental practice and later made a controversial claim that he was the first to make practical use of the gas as an anesthetic, which Colton was always careful to acknowledge. Meeting at another lecture in 1863 in New Haven, Conn., J.H. Smith, a dentist, and Colton extracted more than a thousand teeth in less than a month while using the anesthetic.

Colton, with John Allen, established the Colton Dental Association, which was an immensely successful painless tooth-extraction service. The New York City-based organization opened branch offices in six other cities. In addition to his work with anesthesia, Colton invented an electric motor, which was exhibited in 1847. After moving to California during the Gold Rush days, he practiced medicine there for a short time and was then appointed a justice of the peace in San Francisco.

CARLOS J. FINLAY
(b. Dec. 3, 1833, Puerto Príncipe, Cuba—d. Aug. 20, 1915, Havana)

Cuban epidemiologist Carlos J. Finlay discovered that yellow fever is transmitted from infected to healthy humans by a mosquito. Although he published experimental evidence of this discovery in 1886, his ideas were ignored for 20 years.

A graduate of Jefferson Medical College, Philadelphia (1855), he returned to Cuba, where he practiced medicine in Matanzas and Havana. In 1879 Finlay was appointed by the Cuban government to work with the North American commission studying the causes of yellow fever, and two years later he was chosen to attend the fifth International Sanitary Conference in Washington, D.C., as the Cuban delegate. At the conference, Finlay urged the study of yellow fever vectors, and soon afterward he stated that the carrier was the mosquito *Culex fasciatus*, now known as *Aedes aegypti*.

In 1900 the U.S. Army Yellow Fever Board, which was headed by the physician Walter Reed, arrived in Cuba, and Finlay attempted to persuade Reed of his mosquito-vector theory. Although skeptical, Reed decided to investigate the idea, refining Finlay's experimental procedures in the process. Reed's proof that mosquitoes do indeed transmit yellow fever (1900) and William Gorgas' eradication of the disease in Cuba and Panama followed. Finlay was appointed chief sanitation officer of Cuba (1902–09), and after his death the Finlay Institute for Investigations in Tropical Medicine was created in his honour by the Cuban government.

FRIEDRICH GUSTAV JACOB HENLE
(b. July 19, 1809, Fürth, Bavaria [Germany]—d. May 13, 1885, Göttingen, Ger.)

German pathologist Friedrich Gustav Jacob Henle is one of history's outstanding anatomists. His influence on the development of histology is comparable to the effect on gross anatomy of the work of the Renaissance master Andreas Vesalius.

While a student of the German physiologist Johannes Müller at the universities of Bonn (M.D., 1832) and Berlin (1832–34), Henle published the first descriptions of the structure and distribution of human epithelial tissue and of the fine structures of the eye and brain. In his paper "Von den Miasmen und Contagien und von den miasmatisch-contagiösen Krankheiten" (1840; "On Miasmas and Contagions and on the Miasmatic-Contagious Diseases"), he embraced the unpopular microorganism theory of contagion put forth by the Renaissance forerunner of modern epidemiology, Girolamo Fracastoro, stating, "The material of contagions is not only an organic but a *living* one and is indeed endowed with a life of its own, which is, in relation to the diseased body, a *parasitic organism.*"

While professor of anatomy (1840–44) at the University of Zürich, he published his *Allgemeine Anatomie* (1841; "General Anatomy"), the first systematic treatise of histology, followed by the *Handbuch der rationellen Pathologie,* 2 vol. (1846–53; "Handbook of Rational Pathology"), written while he was professor of anatomy and pathology at the University of Heidelberg (1844–52). The *Handbuch,* describing diseased organs in relation to their normal physiological functions, represents the beginning of modern pathology. Among his students at the University of Göttingen (1852–85) was Robert Koch, who brought Henle's belief in a germ theory to fruition.

SIR PATRICK MANSON
(b. Oct. 3, 1844, Old Meldrum, Aberdeen, Scot.—d. April 9, 1922, London, Eng.)

British parasitologist Sir Patrick Manson founded the field of tropical medicine. He was the first to discover (1877–79) that an insect (mosquito) can be host to a developing parasite (the worm *Filaria bancrofti*) that is the cause of a human disease (filariasis, which occurs when the worms invade body tissues). His research, and Alphonse Laveran's discovery of the malarial parasite, facilitated Sir Ronald Ross's elucidation of the transmission of malaria by mosquitoes.

From 1866 to 1889 Manson practiced medicine in Hong Kong and other coastal Chinese cities, where he was one of the first to introduce vaccination. He instituted the Medical School of Hong Kong, which developed later (1911) into the University of Hong Kong. In 1890 he settled in London, where he organized the London School of Tropical Medicine (1899). He was knighted in 1903 and continued to practice medicine until his death. His textbook *Tropical Diseases* (1898) became a standard work.

WILLIAM THOMAS MORTON
(b. Aug. 9, 1819, Charlton, Mass., U.S.—d. July 15, 1868, New York City)

American dental surgeon William Thomas Morton in 1846 gave the first successful public demonstration of ether anesthesia during surgery. He is credited with gaining the medical world's acceptance of surgical anesthesia.

Morton began dental practice in Boston in 1844. In January 1845 he was present at Massachusetts General Hospital, Boston, when Horace Wells, his former dental partner, attempted unsuccessfully to demonstrate the anodyne properties of nitrous oxide gas. Determined to find a more reliable pain-killing chemical, Morton consulted his former teacher, Boston chemist Charles Jackson, with whom he had previously done work on pain relief. The two discussed the use of ether, and Morton first used it in extraction of a tooth on Sept. 30, 1846. On October 16 he successfully demonstrated its use, administering ether to a patient undergoing a tumour operation in the same theatre where Wells had failed nearly two years earlier.

Unfortunately, Morton attempted to obtain exclusive rights to the use of ether anesthesia. He spent the remainder of his life engaged in a costly contention with Jackson, who claimed priority in the discovery, despite official recognition accorded to Wells and the rural Georgia physician Crawford Long.

JOHANNES PETER MÜLLER
(b. July 14, 1801, Koblenz, France [of the Consulate]—d. April 28, 1858, Berlin, Ger.)

German physiologist and comparative anatomist Johannes Peter Müller was one of the great natural philosophers of the 19th century. His major work was *Handbuch der Physiologie des Menschen für Vorlesungen*, 2 vol. (1834–40; *Elements of Physiology*).

Müller was the son of a shoemaker. In 1819 he entered the University of Bonn, where the faculty of medicine was permeated with *Naturphilosophie* (philosophy of nature), which the young Müller eagerly espoused. He continued his studies at the University of Berlin, where he came under the influence of the sober, precise anatomist Karl Rudolphi and thereby freed himself from naturalistic speculation.

In 1824 he was granted a lectureship in physiology and comparative anatomy at the University of Bonn. In his inaugural lecture, "Physiology, a science in need of a philosophical view of nature," he outlined his approach to science and maintained that the physiologist must combine empirically established facts with philosophical thinking. Two years later he was appointed associate professor, and in 1830 he became a full professor.

In the meantime, his voluminous *Zur vergleichenden Physiologie des Gesichtssinnes...* (1826; "Comparative Physiology of the Visual Sense...") brought Müller to the attention of scholars by its wealth of new material on human and animal vision. He included the results of analyses of human expressions and research on the compound eyes of insects and crustaceans. His most important achievement, however, was the discovery that each of the sense organs responds to different kinds of stimuli in its own particular way or, as Müller wrote, with its own specific energy. The phenomena of the external world are perceived, therefore, only by the changes they produce in sensory systems. His findings had an impact even on the theory of knowledge.

Müller's monograph "On Imaginary Apparitions" was also published in 1826. According to this theory the eye as a sensory system not only reacts to external optical stimuli but can also be excited by internal stimuli generated by the imagination. Thus, persons who report seeing religious visions, ghosts, or phantoms may actually be experiencing optical sensations and believe them to be of external origin, even though they do not in fact have an adequate external stimulus.

Maintaining an almost incredible level of output at Bonn, he examined many problems in physiology, development, and comparative anatomy. He studied the passage of impulses from afferent nerves (going to the brain and spinal cord) to efferent nerves (going away from the same centres), further elucidating the concept of reflex action. By careful experiments on live frogs, he confirmed the law named after Charles Bell and François Magendie, according to which the anterior roots of the nerves originating from the spinal cord are motor and the posterior roots are sensory. He investigated the nervous system of lower animal species, the intricate structure of glands, and the process of secretion. When tracing the development of the genitalia, he discovered what is now known as the Müllerian duct, which forms the female internal sexual organs. He contributed to knowledge of the composition of the blood and lymph, the process of coagulation, the structure of lymph hearts of frogs, the formation of images on the retina of the eye, and the propagation of sound in the middle ear.

In 1833 Müller was called to Berlin to succeed Rudolphi. In his new post he again carefully explored many problems concerning animal function and structure. His early years in Berlin were devoted mainly to physiology. His *Handbuch der Physiologie des Menschen für Vorlesungen* stimulated further basic research and became a starting point for the mechanistic concept of life processes, which was widely accepted in the second half of the 19th century.

Inspired by the vast Berlin anatomical collection, Müller became interested again in pathology. After the demonstration by his assistant, Theodor Schwann, that the cell was the basic unit of structure in the animal body, he concentrated on the cellular structure of tumours with the aid of a microscope. In 1838 his work

Über den feineren Bau und die Formen der krankhaften Geschwülste (*On the Nature and Structural Characteristics of Cancer, and of Those Morbid Growths Which May Be Confounded with It*) began to establish pathological histology as an independent branch of science. Müller also distinguished himself as a teacher. His students included the renowned physiologist and physicist Hermann Helmholtz and the cellular pathologist Rudolf Virchow.

Beginning in 1840 Müller increasingly focused his research on comparative anatomy and zoology, in so doing becoming one of the most respected scholars in these subjects. He was a master at collecting and classifying specimens. He devised an improved classification of fish and, based on an ingenious analysis of vocal organs, did the same for singing birds. For several years he concentrated on the lowest forms of marine vertebrates, the Cyclostomata and Chondrichthyes. He painstakingly described the structures and complex development of members of various classes of the invertebrate phylum Echinodermata. His last research activities were concerned with the marine protozoans Radiolaria and Foraminifera.

FRANCESCO REDI
(b. Feb. 18, 1626, Arezzo, Italy—d. March 1, 1697, Pisa)

Italian physician and poet Francesco Redi demonstrated that the presence of maggots in putrefying meat does not result from spontaneous generation but from eggs laid on the meat by flies.

He read in the book on generation by William Harvey a speculation that vermin such as insects, worms, and frogs do not arise spontaneously, as was then commonly believed, but from seeds or eggs too small to be seen. In 1668, in one of the first examples of a biological experiment with proper controls, Redi set up a series of flasks containing different meats, half of the flasks sealed, half open. He then repeated the experiment but, instead of sealing the flasks, covered half of them with gauze so that air could enter. Although the meat in all of the flasks putrefied, he found that only in the open and uncovered flasks, which flies had entered freely, did the meat contain maggots. Though correctly concluding that the maggots came from eggs laid on the meat by flies, Redi, surprisingly, still believed that the process of spontaneous generation applied in such cases as gall flies and intestinal worms. Redi is known as a poet chiefly for his *Bacco in Toscana* (1685; "Bacchus in Tuscany").

SIR RONALD ROSS
(b. May 13, 1857, Almora, India—d. Sept. 16, 1932, Putney Heath, London, Eng.)

British doctor Sir Ronald Ross received the Nobel Prize for Physiology or Medicine in 1902 for his work on malaria. His discovery of the malarial parasite in the gastrointestinal tract of the *Anopheles* mosquito led to the realization that malaria was transmitted by *Anopheles* and laid the foundation for combating the disease.

After graduating in medicine (1879), Ross entered the Indian Medical Service and served in the third Anglo-Burmese War (1885). On leave he studied bacteriology in London (1888–89) and then returned to India, where, prompted by Patrick Manson's guidance and assistance, he began (1895) a series of investigations on malaria. He discovered the presence of the malarial parasite within the *Anopheles* mosquito in 1897. Using birds that were sick with malaria, he was soon able to ascertain the entire life cycle of the malarial parasite, including its presence in the mosquito's salivary glands. He demonstrated that malaria is transmitted from infected birds to healthy ones by the bite of a mosquito, a finding that suggested the disease's mode of transmission to humans.

Ross returned to England in 1899 and joined the Liverpool School of Tropical Medicine. He was knighted in 1911. In 1912 he became physician for tropical diseases at King's College Hospital, London, and later director of the Ross Institute and Hospital for Tropical Diseases, founded in his honour. In addition to mathematical papers, poems, and fictional works, he wrote *The Prevention of Malaria* (1910).

SIR JAMES YOUNG SIMPSON
(b. June 7, 1811, Bathgate, Linlithgowshire, Scot.—d. May 6, 1870, London, Eng.)

Scottish obstetrician Sir James Young Simpson was the first to use chloroform in obstetrics and the first in Britain to use ether.

Simpson was professor of obstetrics at the University of Edinburgh, where he obtained his M.D. in 1832. After news of the use of ether in surgery reached Scotland in 1846, Simpson tried it in obstetrics the following January. Later that year he substituted chloroform for ether and published his classic *Account of a New Anaesthetic Agent*.

Simpson persisted in the use of chloroform for relief of labour pains, against opposition of obstetricians and the clergy. He was appointed one of the queen's physicians for Scotland in 1847 and in 1866 was created a baronet. Simpson introduced iron wire sutures and acupressure, a method of arresting hemorrhage, and developed the long obstetrics forceps that are named for him. He is also known for his writings on medical history (especially on leprosy in Scotland) and on fetal pathology and hermaphroditism.

JOHN SNOW
(b. March 15, 1813, York, Yorkshire, Eng.—d. June 16, 1858, London)

English physician John Snow was known for his seminal studies of cholera and is widely viewed as the father of contemporary epidemiology.

By 1836 Snow had begun his formal medical education, eventually receiving a doctor of medicine degree (1844) from the University of London. In 1849 he became a licentiate (licensed specialist) of the Royal College of Physicians of London, rising to an elite level in the medical profession. He lived, conducted research, and maintained a medical practice in the Soho neighbourhood of London.

In 1846 Snow learned of the use of ether in America to relieve pain during surgery. He soon mastered its use, and in 1847 he was appointed as anesthesiologist at St. George's Hospital. Later that year he started working with chloroform. Finding the prevailing drops-in-handkerchief method to be too crude, he developed an apparatus that improved both the safety and the effectiveness of chloroform. His success with administering chloroform to Queen Victoria produced a dramatic increase in the social acceptance of gaseous anesthesia. Snow spoke extensively on his work with anesthetics and wrote the influential book *On Chloroform and Other Anaesthetics*, which was published shortly after his death in 1858.

The first cholera epidemic in London occurred in 1831–32, when Snow was still learning his craft. When the second cholera epidemic occurred, in

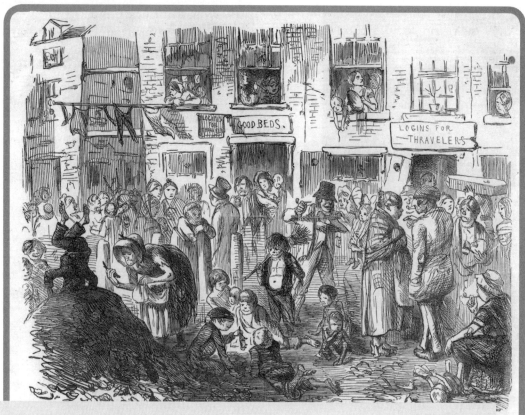

Crowded street scene with children playing among refuse while people pick through it, showing the risk of cholera that comes from unsanitary conditions in slums. Time & Life Pictures/Getty Images

1848–49, he and others founded the London Epidemiological Society, intending to advise the government on ways to combat the disease. Snow reasoned that cholera was caused by a microbelike agent, or germ, that was spread through direct fecal contact, contaminated water, and soiled clothing. However, his theory was at odds with the then prevailing theory that cholera was spread by bad air, or miasma, arising from decayed organic matter. The two etiologic hypotheses—germ theory and miasma—were widely debated, with available clinical and population-based evidence serving as the basis for arguments from both sides. The etiologic debate raged for many years. It was not until the causative organism, *Vibrio cholerae* (initially discovered in 1854), was well characterized in the 1880s that the debate was decided in favour of germ theory.

Snow's respected reputation in epidemiology arose from two classic studies of the third epidemic to reach England, which began in 1853 and lasted until 1855. The first study concerned the Broad Street pump outbreak of 1854, which killed many persons in the Soho neighbourhood. He used skilled reasoning, graphs, and maps to demonstrate the impact of the contaminated water coming from the Broad Street pump. The second study was the "Grand Experiment," also of 1854, which compared London neighbourhoods receiving water from two different companies. One company relied on inlets coming from the upper River Thames, located away from urban pollution, and the other company relied on inlets in the heart of London, where the contamination of water with sewage was common. Snow showed the harmful effect of contaminated water in two nearly equivalent populations, and he suggested intervention strategies to control the epidemic. His ideas and observations, including innovative disease maps, were published in his book *On the Mode of Communication of Cholera* (1855). Later, in the 1930s, Snow's work was republished as a classic work in epidemiology, resulting in lasting recognition of his work.

CHAPTER 4

IMMUNOLOGY AND THE 20TH-CENTURY FIGHT AGAINST INFECTIOUS DISEASE

The 20th century produced such a plethora of discoveries and advances that medicine was fundamentally changed. In 1901, for instance, in the United Kingdom the expectation of life at birth, a primary indicator of the effect of health care on mortality (but also reflecting the state of health education, housing, and nutrition), was 48 years for males and 51.6 years for females. After steady increases, by the 1980s life expectancy had reached 71.4 years for males and 77.2 years for females. Other industrialized nations showed similar dramatic increases. Indeed, the outlook was so altered that, with the exception of diseases such as cancer and AIDS (acquired immunodeficiency syndrome), attention became focused on morbidity rather than mortality, and the emphasis changed from keeping people alive to keeping them fit.

The rapid progress of medicine in this era was reinforced by enormous improvements in communication between scientists throughout the world. Through publications, conferences, and—later—computers and electronic media, they freely exchanged ideas and reported on their endeavours. No longer was it common for an individual to work in isolation. Although specialization increased, teamwork became the norm. It consequently became more difficult to ascribe medical accomplishments to particular individuals.

In the first half of the century, emphasis continued to be placed on combating infection, and notable landmarks were also attained in endocrinology, nutrition, and other areas. In the years following World War II, insights derived from cell biology altered basic concepts of the disease process; new discoveries in biochemistry and physiology opened the way for more precise diagnostic tests and more effective therapies; and spectacular advances in biomedical engineering enabled the physician and surgeon to probe into the structures and functions of the body by noninvasive imaging techniques like ultrasound (sonar), computerized axial tomography (CAT), and nuclear magnetic resonance (NMR). With each new scientific development, medical practices of just a few years earlier became obsolete.

INFECTIOUS DISEASES AND CHEMOTHERAPY

In the years following the turn of the century, ongoing research concentrated on the nature of infectious diseases and their means of transmission. Increasing numbers of pathogenic organisms were discovered and classified. Some, such as the rickettsias, which cause diseases like typhus, were smaller than bacteria, whereas some were larger, such as the protozoans that engender malaria and other tropical diseases. The smallest to be identified were the viruses, producers of many diseases, among them mumps, measles, German measles, and poliomyelitis. In 1910 Peyton Rous showed that a virus could also cause a malignant tumour, a sarcoma in chickens. There was still little to be done, however, for the victims of most infectious organisms. Indeed, drainage, poultices, and ointments in the case of local infections and rest and nourishment for severe diseases remained the primary means of treatment. Thus, the search for new treatments, primarily in the form of chemical agents, was of utmost importance.

Germany was well to the forefront in medical progress. The scientific approach to medicine had been developed there long before it spread to other countries, and postgraduates flocked to German medical schools from all over the world. The opening decade of the 20th century has been well described as the golden age of German medicine. Outstanding among its leaders was Paul Ehrlich, who experimented with the effects of various chemical substances on disease organisms. In 1910, with his colleague Sahachiro Hata, he conducted tests on arsphenamine, once sold under the commercial name Salvarsan. Their success inaugurated the chemotherapeutic era, which was to revolutionize the treatment and control of infectious diseases. Salvarsan, a synthetic preparation containing arsenic, is lethal to the microorganism responsible for syphilis. Until the introduction of penicillin, Salvarsan or one of its modifications remained the standard treatment of syphilis and went far toward bringing this social and medical scourge under control.

THE INTRODUCTION OF ANTIBIOTICS

Since their discovery in the early 20th century, antibiotics have revolutionized the treatment of bacterial diseases. Some of the first antibiotics to come into use included Prontosil and penicillin. Penicillin and many other antibiotics are natural microbial products, but chemists also are able to modify the structures of many of these products to generate semisynthetic and even wholly synthetic antibiotics. Prontosil is an example of a synthetic antibacterial agent.

SULFONAMIDE DRUGS

In 1932 the German bacteriologist Gerhard Domagk announced that the red dye Prontosil is active against streptococcal infections in mice and humans. Soon afterward French workers showed that its active antibacterial agent is sulfanilamide. In 1936 the English physician Leonard Colebrook and his colleagues provided

SULFONAMIDE

Sulfonamides are compounds characterized chemically as the amides of sulfonic acids. The class includes several groups of drugs used in the treatment of bacterial infections, diabetes mellitus, edema, hypertension, and gout.

The bacteriostatic sulfonamide drugs, often called sulfa drugs, include sulfanilamide and numerous compounds closely related to it. Other groups of sulfonamide drugs have been developed by exploiting observations made during clinical evaluation of sulfanilamide derivatives. Examples of these drugs are probenecid, introduced as an agent for intensifying the action of penicillin but now principally used in treating gout; acetazolamide and furosemide, which are diuretics; and tolbutamide, a hypoglycemic. Chlorothiazide and hydrochlorothiazide are effective both as diuretics and in reducing blood pressure.

The first sulfonamide drug, introduced in 1932, was a red azo dye called Prontosil. As new sulfonamides were synthesized, more effective and less toxic agents were discovered. Some, which are not absorbed, can be administered orally to treat specific localized infections in the gastrointestinal tract. Others are absorbed slowly or excreted slowly and therefore are longer acting.

Sulfonamides are oily liquids or crystalline solids that are almost always prepared by the reaction of a sulfonyl chloride with ammonia or an amine, most commonly in the presence of caustic alkali. All the sulfonamides are capable of causing drug intoxication (poisoning), and some patients are hypersensitive to them. The most common side effects are nausea, vomiting, and mental confusion. The signs of hypersensitivity are fever and skin eruptions. Signs of intoxication include anemia, which results from destruction of red blood cells, and leukopenia, which results from the destruction of white blood cells. Irritation of the kidneys and obstruction of the free flow of urine are undesirable reactions that can be prevented.

overwhelming evidence of the efficacy of both Prontosil and sulfanilamide in streptococcal septicemia (bloodstream infection), thereby ushering in the sulfonamide era. New sulfonamides, which appeared with astonishing rapidity, had greater potency, wider antibacterial range, or lower toxicity. Some stood the test of time, whereas others, like the original sulfanilamide and its immediate successor, sulfapyridine, were replaced by safer and more powerful successors.

Penicillin

A dramatic episode in medical history occurred in 1928, when Alexander Fleming noticed the inhibitory action of a stray mold on a plate culture of staphylococcus bacteria in his laboratory at St. Mary's Hospital, London. Many other bacteriologists must have made the observation, but none had realized the possible implications. The mold was a strain of *Penicillium—P. notatum—*which gave its name to the now-famous drug penicillin. In spite of his conviction that penicillin was a potent antibacterial agent, Fleming was unable to carry his work to fruition, mainly because biochemists at the time were unable to isolate it in sufficient quantities or in a sufficiently pure form to allow its use on patients.

Ten years later Howard Florey, Ernst Chain, and their colleagues at Oxford University took up the problem again. They isolated penicillin in a form that was fairly pure (by standards then current)

and demonstrated its potency and relative lack of toxicity. By then World War II had begun, and techniques to facilitate commercial production were developed in the United States. By 1944 adequate amounts were available to meet the extraordinary needs of wartime.

Antituberculous Drugs

While penicillin is the most useful and the safest antibiotic, it suffers from certain disadvantages. One of the most important of these is that it is not active against *Mycobacterium tuberculosis*, the bacillus of tuberculosis. In view of the importance of tuberculosis as a public health hazard, this is a serious defect. The position was rapidly rectified when, in 1944, Selman Waksman, Albert Schatz, and Elizabeth Bugie announced the discovery of streptomycin from cultures of a soil organism, *Streptomyces griseus*, and stated that it was active against *M. tuberculosis*. Subsequent clinical trials amply confirmed this claim. Streptomycin suffers, however, from the great disadvantage that the tubercle bacillus tends to become resistant to it. Fortunately, other drugs became available to supplement it, the two most important being para-aminosalicylic acid (PAS) and isoniazid. With a combination of two or more of these preparations, the outlook in tuberculosis improved immeasurably. The disease was not conquered, but it was brought well under control in the latter part of the 20th century.

OTHER ANTIBIOTICS

In addition to its inactivity against *M. tuberculosis*, penicillin is also ineffective against certain other types of microorganisms pathogenic to humans. During the 1950s the search for antibiotics to fill this gap resulted in a steady stream of them, some with a much wider antibacterial range than penicillin (the so-called broad-spectrum antibiotics) and some capable of coping with those microorganisms that are inherently resistant to penicillin or that have developed resistance through exposure to penicillin.

This tendency of microorganisms to develop resistance to penicillin at one time threatened to become almost as serious a problem as the development of resistance to streptomycin by the bacillus of tuberculosis. Fortunately, early appreciation of the problem by clinicians resulted in more discriminate use of penicillin. Scientists continued to look for means of obtaining new varieties of penicillin, and their researches produced the so-called semisynthetic antibiotics, some of which are active when taken by mouth, while others are effective against microorganisms that have developed resistance to the earlier form of penicillin.

IMMUNOLOGY AND IMMUNIZATION

Dramatic though they undoubtedly were, the advances in chemotherapy still left one important area vulnerable, that of the viruses. It was in bringing viruses under control that advances in immunology—the study of immunity—played such a striking part. One of the paradoxes of medicine is that the first large-scale immunization against a viral disease was instituted and established long before viruses were discovered. When Edward Jenner introduced vaccination against the virus that causes smallpox, the identification of viruses was still 100 years in the future, and it took almost another half century to discover an effective method of producing antiviral vaccines that were both safe and effective.

In the meantime, however, the process by which the body reacts against infectious organisms to generate immunity became better understood. In Paris, Élie Metchnikoff had already detected the role of white blood cells in the immune reaction, and Jules Bordet had identified antibodies in the blood serum. The mechanisms of antibody activity were used to devise diagnostic tests for a number of diseases. In 1906 August von Wassermann gave his name to the blood test for syphilis, and in 1908 the tuberculin test—the skin test for tuberculosis—came into use.

ANTIBACTERIAL VACCINATION

At the same time that methods for antibody detection were developed for the diagnosis of bacterial infection, methods of producing effective substances for inoculation were improved, and immunization against bacterial diseases made rapid progress. This work was supported by the continued effort to identify and characterize infectious organisms.

TYPHOID VACCINE

In 1897 English bacteriologist Almroth Wright introduced a vaccine prepared from killed typhoid bacilli as a preventive of typhoid. Preliminary trials in the Indian army produced excellent results, and typhoid vaccination was adopted for the use of British troops serving in the South African War. Unfortunately, the method of administration was inadequately controlled, and the government sanctioned inoculations only for soldiers that "voluntarily presented themselves for this purpose prior to their embarkation for the seat of war." The result was that, according to the official records, only 14,626 men volunteered out of a total strength of 328,244 who served during the three years of the war. Although later analysis showed that inoculation had had a beneficial effect, there were 57,684 cases of typhoid—approximately

TYPHOID MARY

(b. 1870?—d. Nov. 11, 1938, North Brother Island, New York, N.Y., U.S.)

Typhoid Mary was the byname of Mary Mallon, the typhoid carrier who allegedly gave rise to the most famous outbreaks of carrier-borne disease in medical history.

Mary was first recognized as a carrier of the typhoid bacteria during an epidemic of typhoid fever in 1904 that spread through Oyster Bay, New York, where she worked as a cook. By the time the disease had been traced to its source in a household where she had recently been employed, Mary had disappeared. She continued to work as a cook, moving from household to household, until 1907, when she resurfaced, working in a Park Avenue home in Manhattan.

Again Mary fled, but authorities led by George Soper, a sanitary engineer in the New York City Department of Health, finally overtook her and had her committed to an isolation centre on North Brother Island, off the Bronx, New York. There she stayed, despite an appeal to the U.S. Supreme Court, until 1910, when the health department released her on condition that she never accept employment that involved the handling of food.

Four years later, Soper began looking for Mary again when an epidemic broke out at a sanatorium in Newfoundland, New Jersey, and at Sloane Maternity Hospital in Manhattan, New York. Mary had worked as a cook at both places. She was at last found in a suburban home in Westchester county, New York, and was returned to North Brother Island, where she remained the rest of her life. A paralytic stroke in 1932 led to her slow death, six years later.

Mary's claim to having been born in the United States was never confirmed, nor was her age ever verified. Fifty-one original cases of typhoid and three deaths were directly attributed to her (countless more were indirectly attributed), although she herself was immune to the typhoid bacillus (Salmonella typhi).

one in six of the British troops engaged—with 9,022 deaths.

A bitter controversy over the merits of the vaccine followed, but before the outbreak of World War I immunization had been officially adopted by the army. Comparative statistics would seem to provide striking confirmation of the value of antityphoid inoculation, even allowing for the better sanitary arrangements in the latter war. In the South African War the annual incidence of enteric infections (typhoid and paratyphoid) was 105 per 1,000 troops, and the annual death rate was 14.6 per 1,000. The comparable figures for World War I were 2.35 and 0.139, respectively.

It was perhaps a sign of the increasingly critical outlook that developed in medicine in the post-1945 era that experts continued to differ on some aspects of typhoid immunization. There was no question as to its fundamental efficacy, but there was considerable variation of opinion as to the best vaccine to use and the most effective way of administering it. Moreover, it was often difficult to decide to what extent the decline in typhoid was attributable to improved sanitary conditions and what to the greater use of the vaccine.

TETANUS VACCINE

The other great hazard of war that was brought under control in World War I was tetanus. This was achieved by the prophylactic injection of tetanus antitoxin into all wounded men. The serum was originally prepared by the bacteriologists Emil von Behring and Kitasato Shibasaburo in 1890–92, and the results of this first large-scale trial amply confirmed its efficacy. (Tetanus antitoxin is a sterile solution of antibody globulins—a type of blood protein—from immunized horses or cattle.)

It was not until the 1930s, however, that an efficient vaccine, or toxoid, as it is known in the cases of tetanus and diphtheria, was produced against tetanus. (Tetanus toxoid is a preparation of the toxin—or poison—produced by the microorganism; injected into humans, it stimulates the body's own defenses against the disease, thus bringing about immunity.) Again, a war was to provide the opportunity for testing on a large scale, and experience with tetanus toxoid in World War II indicated that it gave a high degree of protection.

DIPHTHERIA VACCINE

The story of diphtheria is comparable to that of tetanus, though even more dramatic. First, as with tetanus antitoxin, came the preparation of diphtheria antitoxin by Behring and Kitasato in 1890. As the antitoxin came into general use for the treatment of cases, the death rate began to decline. There was no significant fall in the number of cases, however, until a toxin–antitoxin mixture, introduced by Behring in 1913, was used to immunize children. A more effective toxoid was introduced by the French bacteriologist Gaston Ramon in 1923, and with subsequent improvements this became one of the most effective vaccines available in medicine. Where mass immunization of children with the toxoid was practiced, as in the United States and Canada beginning in the late 1930s and in England and Wales in the early 1940s, cases of diphtheria and deaths from the disease became almost nonexistent. In England and Wales, for instance, the number of deaths fell from an annual average of 1,830 in 1940–44 to zero in 1969. Administration of a combined vaccine against diphtheria, pertussis (whooping cough), and tetanus (DPT) is recommended for young children. Although an increasing number of dangerous side effects from the DPT vaccine have been reported, it continues to be used in most countries because of the protection it affords.

BCG Vaccine for Tuberculosis

If, as is universally accepted, prevention is better than cure, immunization is the ideal way of dealing with diseases caused by microorganisms. An effective, safe vaccine protects the individual from disease, whereas chemotherapy merely copes with the infection once the individual has been affected. In spite of its undoubted value, however, immunization has been a recurring source of dispute. Like vaccination against typhoid (and against poliomyelitis later), tuberculosis immunization evoked widespread contention.

In 1908 Albert Calmette, a pupil of Pasteur, and Camille Guérin produced an avirulent (weakened) strain of the tubercle bacillus. About 13 years later, vaccination of children against tuberculosis was introduced, with a vaccine made from this avirulent strain and known as BCG (bacillus Calmette-Guérin) vaccine. Although it was adopted in France, Scandinavia, and elsewhere, British and U.S. authorities frowned upon its use on the grounds that it was not safe and that the statistical evidence in its favour was not convincing.

One of the stumbling blocks in the way of its widespread adoption was what came to be known as the Lübeck disaster. In the spring of 1930, 249 infants were vaccinated with BCG vaccine in Lübeck, Ger., and by autumn, 73 of the 249 were dead. Criminal proceedings were instituted against those responsible for giving the vaccine. The final verdict was that the vaccine had been contaminated, and the BCG vaccine itself was exonerated from any responsibility for the deaths. A bitter controversy followed, but in the end the protagonists of the vaccine won when a further trial showed that the vaccine was safe and that it protected four out of five of those vaccinated.

Immunization Against Viral Diseases

With the exception of smallpox, it was not until well into the 20th century that efficient viral vaccines became available. In fact, it was not until the 1930s that much began to be known about viruses. The two developments that contributed most to the rapid growth in knowledge after that time were the introduction of tissue culture as a means of growing viruses in the laboratory and the availability of the electron microscope. Once the virus could be cultivated with comparative ease in the laboratory, the research worker could study it with care and evolve methods for producing one of the two requirements for a safe and effective vaccine: either a virus that was so attenuated, or weakened, that it could not produce the disease for which it was responsible in its normally virulent form; or a killed virus that retained the faculty of inducing a protective antibody response in the vaccinated individual.

The first of the viral vaccines to result from these advances was for yellow fever, developed by the microbiologist Max Theiler in the late 1930s. About 1945 the first relatively effective vaccine was produced for influenza. In 1954 the American physician Jonas E. Salk introduced a vaccine for poliomyelitis, and in 1960 an oral poliomyelitis vaccine, developed by the virologist Albert B. Sabin, came into wide use.

These vaccines went far toward bringing under control three of the major diseases of the time although, in the case of influenza, a major complication is the disturbing proclivity of the virus to change its character from one epidemic to another. Even so, sufficient progress has been made to ensure that a pandemic like the one that swept the world in 1918–19, killing some 25 to 50 million people, is unlikely to occur again. Centres are now equipped to monitor outbreaks of influenza throughout the world in order to establish the identity of the responsible viruses and, if necessary, take steps to produce appropriate vaccines.

During the 1960s effective vaccines came into use for measles and rubella (German measles). Both evoked a certain amount of controversy. In the case of measles in the Western world it was contended that, if acquired in childhood, it is not a particularly hazardous malady, and the naturally acquired disease evokes permanent immunity in the vast majority of cases. Conversely, the vaccine induces a certain number of adverse reactions, and the duration of the immunity it produces is problematical. In the end the official view was that universal measles vaccination is to be commended.

The situation with rubella vaccination was different. This is a fundamentally mild affliction, and the only cause for anxiety is its proclivity to induce congenital deformities if a pregnant woman should acquire the disease. Once an effective vaccine was available, the problem was the extent to which it should be used. Ultimately the consensus was reached that all girls who had not already had the disease should be vaccinated at about 12 years. In the United States children are routinely immunized against measles, mumps, and rubella at the age of 15 months.

THE IMMUNE RESPONSE

With advances in cell biology in the second half of the 20th century came a more profound understanding of both normal and abnormal conditions in the body. Electron microscopy enabled observers to peer more deeply into the structures of the cell, and chemical investigations revealed clues to their functions in the cell's intricate metabolism. The overriding importance of the nuclear genetic material DNA (deoxyribonucleic acid) in regulating the cell's protein and enzyme production lines became evident. A clearer comprehension also emerged of the ways in which the cells of the body defend themselves by modifying their chemical activities to produce antibodies against injurious agents.

Up until the turn of the century, immunity referred mostly to the means of resistance of an animal to invasion by a parasite or microorganism. Around mid-century there arose a growing realization that immunity and immunology cover a much wider field and are concerned with mechanisms for preserving the integrity of the individual. The introduction of organ transplantation, with its dreaded complication of tissue rejection, brought this broader concept of immunology to the fore.

At the same time, research workers and clinicians began to appreciate the far-reaching implications of immunity in relation to endocrinology, genetics, tumour biology, and the biology of a number of other maladies. The so-called autoimmune diseases are caused by an aberrant series of immune responses by which the body's own cells are attacked. Suspicion is growing that a number of major disorders such as diabetes, rheumatoid arthritis, and multiple sclerosis may be caused by similar mechanisms.

In some conditions viruses invade the genetic material of cells and distort their metabolic processes. Such viruses may lie dormant for many years before becoming active. This may be the underlying cause of many cancers, in which cells escape from the usual constraints imposed upon them by the normal body. The dreaded affliction of AIDS is caused by a virus that has a long dormant period and then attacks the cells that produce antibodies. The result is that the affected person is not able to generate an immune response to infections or malignancies.

MAJOR 20TH-CENTURY FIGURES IN IMMUNOLOGY AND INFECTIOUS DISEASE

Many physicians and researchers contributed to the advance of immunology and infectious disease in the 20th century. These individuals frequently came by way of their discoveries through basic research on biochemistry, cells, and microorganisms, with their work leading them to the crossroads of human health and disease. Emil von Behring, Paul Ehrlich, and Selman Waksman are just a few examples of figures whose research fueled progress in these fields.

EMIL VON BEHRING
(b. March 15, 1854, Hansdorf, West
Prussia [now Jankowa Żagańska,
Pol.]—d. March 31, 1917, Marburg, Ger.)

German bacteriologist Emil von Behring
was one of the founders of immunology.
In 1901 he received the first Nobel Prize
for Physiology or Medicine for his work
on serum therapy, particularly for its use
in the treatment of diphtheria.

Behring received his medical degree
in 1878 from the Friedrich-Wilhelms-
Institut, the Prussian army's medical
college, in Berlin. After serving 10 years
with the Army Medical Corps, he became
an assistant (1889) at the Institute for
Hygiene, Berlin, where Robert Koch was
director. There, with the Japanese bacteriologist Kitasato Shibasaburo, he showed
that it was possible to provide an animal
with passive immunity against tetanus
by injecting it with the blood serum of
another animal infected with the disease.
Behring applied this antitoxin (a term
he and Kitasato originated) technique
to achieve immunity against diphtheria.
Administration of diphtheria antitoxin,
developed with Paul Ehrlich and first
successfully marketed in 1892, became a
routine part of the treatment of the disease.

Behring taught at Halle (1894) and
in 1895 moved on to become director of
the Institute of Hygiene at the Philipps
University of Marburg. He became
financially involved with the Farbwerke
Meister, Lucius und Brüning in Höchst,
a dye works that provided laboratories
for his research, which included studies

of tuberculosis. His writings include *Die
praktischen Ziele der Blutserumtherapie*
(1892; "The Practical Goals of Blood
Serum Therapy").

SIR ERNST BORIS CHAIN
(b. June 19, 1906, Berlin, Ger.—d. Aug.
12, 1979, Mulrany, Ire.)

German-born British biochemist Sir Ernst
Boris Chain, with pathologist Howard
Walter Florey (later Baron Florey),
isolated and purified penicillin and
performed the first clinical trials of the
antibiotic. For their pioneering work
on penicillin Chain, Florey, and Sir
Alexander Fleming shared the 1945
Nobel Prize for Physiology or Medicine.

Chain graduated in chemistry and
physiology from the Friedrich Wilhelm
University of Berlin and then engaged
in research at the Institute of Pathology,
Charité Hospital, Berlin (1930–33).
Forced to flee Germany because of the
anti-Semitic policies of Adolf Hitler, he
went first to the University of Cambridge,
working under Sir Frederick G. Hopkins,
and then (1935) to the University of
Oxford, where he worked with Florey on
penicillin.

Chain served as the director of
the International Research Centre
for Chemical Microbiology, Superior
Institute of Health, Rome, from 1948
until 1961. He then joined the faculty of
Imperial College, University of London,
where he was professor of biochemistry
(1961–73), professor emeritus and senior
research fellow (1973–76), and fellow

a cure for puerperal, or childbed, fever, a condition resulting from infection after childbirth or abortion.

Colebrook joined researcher Almroth Wright in 1907 at St. Mary's Hospital. In 1926 Colebrook became interested in the incidence of puerperal fever in women who had just undergone childbirth. Nine years later, he obtained the newly discovered antibacterial drug Prontosil and used it to treat a woman who was dying of puerperal fever. The patient recovered, and the drug was next used successfully on a woman dying of septicemia (blood poisoning). By 1945, as a result of the widespread use of the drug, puerperal fever was no longer a common problem. Prontosil was also used to treat other diseases, including lobar pneumonia.

At the outbreak of World War II, Colebrook went to France to investigate the treatment of burns. He established the efficacy of the sulfonamides and then of penicillin in controlling the infection of burns, urged the wider application of skin-grafting techniques to heal burns, and brought the problem of tissue rejection to the attention of Peter B. Medawar. Colebrook served as director of the Burns Investigation Unit of the Medical Research Council from 1942 to 1948.

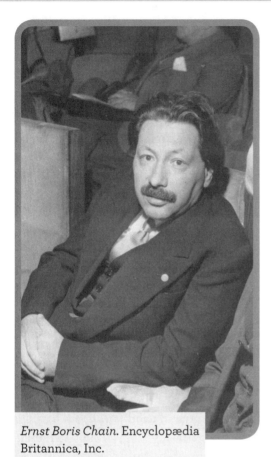
Ernst Boris Chain. Encyclopædia Britannica, Inc.

(1978–79). Chain was knighted in 1969. In addition to his work on antibiotics, Chain studied snake venoms, the spreading factor (an enzyme that facilitates the dispersal of fluids in tissue), and insulin.

Leonard Colebrook
(b. March 2, 1883, Guildford, Surrey, Eng.—d. Sept. 29, 1967, Farnham Common, Buckinghamshire)

English medical researcher Leonard Colebrook introduced the use of Prontosil, the first sulfonamide drug, as

Paul Ehrlich
(b. March 14, 1854, Strehlen, Silesia, Prussia [now Strzelin, Pol.]—d. Aug. 20, 1915, Bad Homburg vor der Höhe, Ger.)

German medical scientist Paul Ehrlich was known for his pioneering work in hematology, immunology, and chemo-therapy and for his discovery of the first effective treatment for syphilis. He received jointly with Élie Metchnikoff the Nobel Prize for Physiology or Medicine in 1908.

After receiving his medical degree from the University of Leipzig in 1878, Ehrlich was offered a position as head physician at the prestigious Charité Hospital in Berlin. There he developed a new staining technique to identify the tuberculosis bacillus (a bacterium) that had been discovered by the German bacteriologist Robert Koch. Ehrlich also differentiated the numerous types of blood cells of the body and thereby laid the foundation for the field of hematology.

While developing new methods for the staining of live tissue, Ehrlich discovered the uses of methylene blue in the treatment of nervous disorders. In other diagnostic advances, he traced a specific chemical reaction in the urine of typhoid patients, tested various medications for reducing or removing fever, and made valuable suggestions for the treatment of eye diseases. Of the 37 scientific contributions that he published between 1879 and 1885, Ehrlich considered the last as the most important: *Das Sauerstoff-Bedürfniss des Organismus* (1885; "The Requirement of the Organism for Oxygen"). In it he established that oxygen consumption varies with different types of tissue and that these variations constitute a measure of the intensity of vital cell processes.

To explain immunological phenomena, Ehrlich developed a hypothesis known as the side-chain theory, which described how antibodies—the protective proteins produced by the immune system—are formed and how they react with other substances. This much-debated hypothesis, although ultimately proven to be incorrect in many particulars, had a profound influence on Ehrlich's later work and on the work of his successors. Thus Ehrlich was able to show experimentally that rabbits subjected to a slow and measured increase of toxic matter were able to survive 5,000 times the fatal dose. In the end, he established precise quantitative patterns of immunity. These findings assumed great importance in 1890, when he met Emil von Behring, who had succeeded in creating an antitoxin against diphtheria. Behring had tried to prepare a serum that could be used in clinical practice, but it was only by adopting Ehrlich's technique of using the blood of live horses that the preparation of a serum of optimum antitoxic effectiveness became possible. Ehrlich developed a way of measuring the effectiveness of serums that was soon adopted all over the world for the standardization of diphtheria serum. He also demonstrated, in 1892, that antibodies are passed in breast milk from mother to newborn.

Ehrlich later began experimenting with the identification and synthesis of substances, not necessarily found in nature, that could kill parasites or inhibit their growth without damaging the

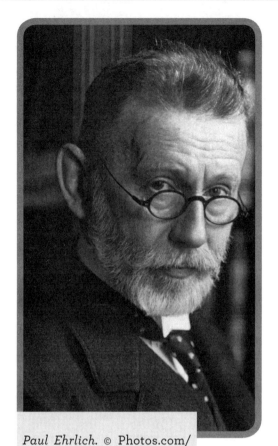

Paul Ehrlich. © Photos.com/ Jupiterimages

content. The first tests, announced in the spring of 1910, proved to be surprisingly successful in the treatment of a whole spectrum of diseases. In the case of yaws, a tropical disease akin to syphilis, a single injection was sufficient. It seemed as if a "magic bullet," to use a favourite expression of Ehrlich's, had been found.

The devastation wrought by syphilis provoked worldwide demand for a new weapon against the disease. Ehrlich, however, would not yet release his discovery for general use, believing as he did that the usual few hundred clinical tests did not suffice in the case of an arsenic preparation, the injection of which required special precautions. In an unheard-of transaction, the manufacturer with whom Ehrlich had collaborated closely, Farbwerke-Hoechst, released a total of 65,000 units gratis to physicians all over the globe.

The greatest distinction bestowed on Ehrlich by the Prussian state was the title "Wirklicher Geheimer Rat," or Privy Councillor, with the predicate of "Exzellenz." Along with numerous other honours, Ehrlich was presented with honorary doctorates by the Universities of Oxford, Chicago, and Athens and an honorary citizenship by Frankfurt am Main, where the institute he founded still bears his name. Having suffered a first stroke in December 1914, Ehrlich succumbed to a second stroke in August of the following year. In its obituary the London *Times* acknowledged Ehrlich's achievement in opening new doors into the unknown, saying, "The whole world is in his debt."

organism. After encountering difficulties with several organisms and compounds, he decided to study the spirochete *Treponema pallidum*, the causal organism of syphilis. Ehrlich had at this time several institutes at his disposal as well as sizable research funds. He also had a staff of highly competent collaborators. In fact, his colleague Hata Sahachirō contributed much to his eventual success in combating syphilis. His preparation 606, later called Salvarsan, was extraordinarily effective and harmless despite its large arsenic

SIR ALEXANDER FLEMING
(b. Aug. 6, 1881, Lochfield Farm, Darvel, Ayrshire, Scot.—d. March 11, 1955, London, Eng.)

Scottish bacteriologist Sir Alexander Fleming was best known for his discovery of penicillin, which marked the beginning of the antibiotic revolution. He shared the 1945 Nobel Prize for Physiology or Medicine with Australian pathologist Howard Walter Florey and British biochemist Ernst Boris Chain, both of whom isolated and purified penicillin.

Fleming began his medical studies in 1901 at St. Mary's Hospital Medical School in London. Although he planned to become a surgeon, a position in the Inoculation Department at St. Mary's Hospital led him to explore the new field of bacteriology instead. There he came under the influence of bacteriologist and immunologist Sir Almroth Edward Wright, whose ideas of vaccine therapy seemed to offer a revolutionary direction in medical treatment.

Between 1909 and 1914, Fleming was a practicing venereologist. During this period, he became one of the first doctors in Britain to administer arsphenamine (Salvarsan). While serving in the Royal Army Medical Corps in World War I, he conducted research on antibacterial substances that would be nontoxic to humans. After the war, Fleming returned to St. Mary's and was promoted to assistant director of the Inoculation Department.

In November 1921 Fleming discovered lysozyme, an enzyme present in body fluids such as saliva and tears that has a mild antiseptic effect. This was the first of his major discoveries. His study of lysozyme, which he considered his best work as a scientist, was a significant contribution to the understanding of how the body fights infection.

On Sept. 3, 1928, shortly after his appointment as professor of bacteriology, Fleming noticed that a culture plate of *Staphylococcus aureus* he had been working on had become contaminated by a fungus. A mold, later identified as *Penicillium notatum* (also called *P. chrysogenum*), had inhibited the growth of the bacteria. He initially called the substance "mould juice" but later named it "penicillin." At first, Fleming thought that he had found an enzyme more potent than lysozyme. He soon realized, however, that penicillin was not an enzyme. Rather, it was an antibiotic—one of the first to be discovered. Fleming knew that penicillin had clinical potential, both as a topical antiseptic and as an injectable antibiotic. However, he failed to stabilize and purify the substance.

Fleming's basic discovery was carried further—in isolating, purifying, testing, and producing penicillin in quantity—because of the work of Florey and Chain. Penicillin eventually came into use during World War II. Fleming was knighted in 1944, and for the last decade of his life, he was celebrated for his discovery of penicillin. He acted as a world ambassador for medicine and science. Initially a shy, uncommunicative man and a poor lecturer, he blossomed under the attention he received, becoming one of the world's best-known scientists.

HOWARD WALTER FLOREY
(b. Sept. 24, 1898, Adelaide, Austl.—d. Feb. 21, 1968, Oxford, Eng.)

Australian pathologist Howard Florey, with Ernst Boris Chain, isolated and purified penicillin for general clinical use. For this research Florey, Chain, and Sir Alexander Fleming shared the Nobel Prize for Physiology or Medicine in 1945.

Florey studied medicine at Adelaide and Oxford universities until 1924. After holding teaching and research posts at Cambridge and Sheffield universities, he was professor of pathology at Oxford (1935–62). He was appointed provost of Queen's College, Oxford (1962), and chancellor of the Australian National University, Canberra (1965), positions he held until his death. He also served as president of the Royal Society (1960–65). He was knighted in 1944 and made life peer, assuming his title as baron, in 1965. Florey investigated tissue inflammation and secretion of mucous membranes. He succeeded in purifying lysozyme, a bacteria-destroying enzyme originally discovered by Fleming. Florey characterized the substances acted upon by the enzyme. In 1939 he surveyed other naturally occurring antibacterial substances, concentrating on penicillin. With Chain and others, he demonstrated its curative properties in human studies and developed methods for its production.

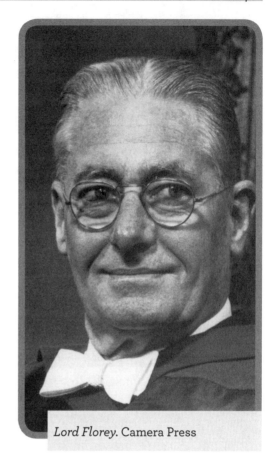

Lord Florey. Camera Press

Following World War II and the work of his research team in North Africa, penicillin came into widespread clinical use.

CAMILLE GUÉRIN
(b. Dec. 22, 1872, Poitiers, France—d. June 9, 1961, Paris)

French scientist Camille Guérin, with Albert Calmette, developed the BCG (Bacillus Calmette-Guérin) vaccine, which became widely used in Europe and America in combatting tuberculosis.

After preparing for a career in veterinary medicine, Guérin joined Calmette at the Pasteur Institute in Lille in 1897; from that time on he devoted his life to vaccination research. As early as 1906 he demonstrated that resistance to tuberculosis was related to the presence in the body of living bacilli. For a period of 13 years Calmette and Guérin produced increasingly less virulent subcultures of a bovine strain of the tubercle bacillus. In 1921 the two researchers believed the bacillus they had produced was harmless to humans but retained its power to stimulate antibody formation. In 1922 they first used it to vaccinate newborn infants at the Charité Hospital in Paris.

From the 1930s, after all questions about its use were resolved, mass vaccination programs were carried out in Japan, Russia, China, England, Canada, France, and other countries. In 1950 the University of Illinois and the Research Foundation were licensed to prepare, distribute, and sell the vaccine in the United States. At the time of his death, Guérin was honorary director of the Pasteur Institute.

KITASATO SHIBASABURO
(b. Jan. 29, 1853, Kitanosato, Higo province [now Kumamoto prefecture], Japan—d. June 13, 1931, Tokyo)

Japanese physician and bacteriologist Kitasato Shibasaburo (also spelled Kitazato Shibasaburō) helped discover a method to prevent tetanus and diphtheria and, in the same year as Alexandre Yersin, discovered the infectious agent responsible for the bubonic plague.

Kitasato began his study of medicine at Igakusho Hospital (now Kumamoto Medical School). When his mentor, Dutch physician C. G. van Mansvelt, left the school, Kitasato entered Tokyo Medical School (now the Faculty of Medicine, University of Tokyo). After graduation (M.D., 1883) he carried out bacteriological research at the Central Sanitary Bureau of the Ministry of Home Affairs.

In 1885 Kitasato moved to Berlin to join the laboratory of German bacteriologist Robert Koch. There, with Emil von Behring, he studied tetanus and diphtheria, two bacterial infections that cause symptoms through the secretion of toxins. In 1889 Kitasato succeeded in obtaining the first pure culture of the tetanus bacteria (bacilli), and the following year he and von Behring demonstrated that immunity to tetanus could be achieved by injecting a susceptible animal with serum containing antitoxin produced in the blood of an animal exposed to the bacterial toxin. They soon successfully applied this approach, called serum therapy, to the treatment of diphtheria.

Returning to Japan in 1892, Kitasato founded and became president of the Institute for Infectious Diseases, a laboratory near Tokyo that was incorporated in 1899 into the Ministry of Home Affairs. The next year he founded Yojoen, a sanatorium for victims of tuberculosis, and concurrently served as president of both organizations.

Kitasato was sent to Hong Kong in 1894 to investigate an outbreak of the bubonic plague. Within a month he identified the causative organism of the plague, the bacillus *Pasteurella pestis* (now called *Yersinia pestis*; renamed after French bacteriologist Alexandre Yersin, who independently discovered the plague bacillus during the Hong Kong epidemic).

In 1914 Kitasato resigned the directorship of the imperial institute and founded the Kitasato Institute. He became the first dean of the medical school of Keio University, an institution he helped establish, in 1917 and held this position until 1928. When the Japanese Medical Association was founded in 1923, he became its first president. In 1924 the emperor invested him with the title of baron.

ALBERT BRUCE SABIN
(b. Aug. 26, 1906, Białystok, Poland, Russian Empire—d. March 3, 1993, Washington, D.C., U.S.)

Polish American physician and microbiologist Albert Bruce Sabin was best known for developing the oral polio vaccine. He was also known for his research in the fields of human viral diseases, toxoplasmosis, and cancer.

Sabin immigrated with his parents to the United States in 1921 and became an American citizen nine years later. He received an M.D. degree from New York University in 1931, where he began research on human poliomyelitis. After serving for two years as a house physician at Bellevue Hospital in New York City, he attended the Lister Institute of Preventive Medicine in London. In 1935 he joined the staff of the Rockefeller Institute for Medical Research in New York City, where he was the first researcher to demonstrate the growth of poliovirus in human nervous tissue outside the body.

In 1939 Sabin became associate professor of pediatrics at the University of Cincinnati College of Medicine in Ohio and chief of the division of infectious diseases at the Children's Hospital Research Foundation of the college. He later became professor of research pediatrics. While at the college, he disproved the prevailing theory that the poliovirus enters the body through the nose and respiratory system; he subsequently demonstrated that human poliomyelitis is primarily an infection of the digestive tract.

Sabin postulated that live, weakened (attenuated) virus, administered orally, would provide immunity over a longer period of time than killed, injected virus. By 1957 he had isolated strains of each of the three types of poliovirus that were not strong enough to produce the disease itself but were capable of stimulating the production of antibodies. He then proceeded to conduct preliminary experiments in the oral administration of these attenuated strains. Cooperative studies were conducted with scientists from Mexico, the Netherlands, and the Soviet Union, and finally, in extensive field trials on children, the effectiveness of the new vaccine was conclusively demonstrated. The Sabin oral polio vaccine was approved for use in the United States in 1960 and became the main defense against polio throughout the world.

Sabin also isolated the B virus, conducted research that led to the development of vaccines for sandfly fever and dengue, studied how immunity to viruses is developed, investigated viruses that affect the nervous system, and studied the role of viruses in cancer. Sabin became professor emeritus at Cincinnati in 1971, and from 1974 to 1982 he was a research professor at the Medical University of South Carolina in Charleston.

JONAS EDWARD SALK
(b. Oct. 28, 1914, New York, N.Y., U.S.—d. June 23, 1995, La Jolla, Calif.)

American physician and medical researcher Jonas Edward Salk showed that killed poliovirus could induce antibody formation without producing disease. This discovery led him to develop the first safe and effective vaccine for polio.

Salk received his M.D. in 1939 from New York University (NYU) College of Medicine. In 1942 he went to the University of Michigan School of Public Health, where he joined Thomas Francis, Jr. Salk had met Francis at NYU, where the latter had conducted his initial studies of killed-virus immunology.

In 1947 Salk moved to Pittsburgh, having accepted a position as associate professor of bacteriology and head of the Virus Research Laboratory at the University of Pittsburgh School of Medicine. There he began research on polio, an acute viral infectious disease of the nervous system. The disease struck hundreds of thousands of children annually in the mid-20th century and was widely feared because of its ability to cause permanent paralysis of muscles in the limbs, chest, or throat. Salk worked with scientists from other universities to classify the various strains of poliovirus, and he corroborated other studies in identifying three separate strains. He then demonstrated that killed virus of each of the three, although incapable of producing the disease, could induce antibody formation in monkeys.

In 1952 he conducted field tests of his killed-virus vaccine, first on children who had recovered from polio and then on subjects who had not had the disease. The tests were successful in that the children's antibody levels rose significantly and no subjects contracted polio from the vaccine. In 1954 Francis conducted a mass field trial, and the vaccine, injected by needle, was found to safely reduce the incidence of polio. On April 12, 1955, the vaccine was released for use in the United States. In the following years the incidence of polio in the United States fell dramatically. In the 1960s Albert Sabin introduced his polio vaccine, known as oral poliovirus vaccine (OPV) or Sabin vaccine. This vaccine differed from Salk's in that it contained live attenuated (weakened) virus and was given orally.

SELMAN WAKSMAN
(b. July 22, 1888, Priluka, Ukraine, Russian Empire [now Pryluky, Ukraine]—d. Aug. 16, 1973, Hyannis, Mass., U.S.)

Ukrainian-born American biochemist Selman Abraham Waksman was one of the world's foremost authorities on soil microbiology. After the discovery of penicillin, he played a major role in initiating a calculated, systematic search for antibiotics among microbes. His consequent codiscovery of the antibiotic streptomycin, the first specific agent effective in the treatment of tuberculosis, brought him the 1952 Nobel Prize for Physiology or Medicine.

A naturalized U.S. citizen (1916), Waksman spent most of his career at Rutgers University, New Brunswick, New Jersey, where he served as professor of soil microbiology (1930–40), professor of microbiology and chairman of the department (1940–58), and director of the Rutgers Institute of Microbiology (1949–58). During his extensive study of the actinomycetes (filamentous, bacteria-like microorganisms found in the soil), he extracted from them antibiotics (a term he coined in 1941) valuable for their killing effect not only on gram-positive bacteria, against which penicillin is effective, but also on gram-negative bacteria, of which the tubercle bacillus (*Mycobacterium tuberculosis*) is one.

In 1940 Waksman, along with Albert Schatz and Elizabeth Bugie, isolated actinomycin from soil bacteria but found it to be extremely toxic when given to test animals. Three years later they extracted the relatively nontoxic streptomycin from the actinomycete *Streptomyces griseus* and found that it exercised repressive influence on tuberculosis. In combination with other chemotherapeutic agents, streptomycin has become a major factor in controlling the disease. Waksman also isolated and developed several other antibiotics, including neomycin, that have been used in treating many infectious diseases of humans, domestic animals, and plants. Among Waksman's books are *Principles of Soil Microbiology* (1927), regarded as one of the most exhaustive works on the subject, and *My Life with the Microbes* (1954), an autobiography.

CHAPTER 5

PROGRESS IN THE UNDERSTANDING OF DISEASE IN THE 20TH CENTURY

In the 20th century there occurred rapid growth and progress in the understanding of disease. Medical and scientific literature expanded greatly, resulting in a voluminous collection of journals and texts devoted solely to the better understanding of human disease. Much of this progress related to improvements in scientists' knowledge of hormones and other biomolecules, thereby giving rise to the field of endocrinology. Two of the most significant discoveries in this new field were the isolation and subsequent characterization of the role of insulin in diabetes mellitus and the invention of the contraceptive pill as a form of birth control. Paralleling these advances were discoveries in the areas of nutrition and metabolism—the utilization and breakdown of nutrients by the body.

Another area of medicine that became firmly established in the 20th century was tropical medicine, which is concerned with diseases that occur primarily in countries with tropical or subtropical climates. This field of medicine emerged as a vital area of public health because of the destructive social and economic effects of tropical diseases, such as malaria and leprosy. Despite the emergence of tropical medicine, however, tropical diseases remain one of the largest public health concerns in the 21st century. Indeed, annual cases of malaria worldwide are estimated at 250 million, with roughly 900,000 deaths resulting—most of them young children in Africa.

ENDOCRINOLOGY

At the beginning of the 20th century, endocrinology was in its infancy. Indeed, it was not until 1905 that Ernest H. Starling, one of the many brilliant pupils of Edward Sharpey-Schafer, the dean of British physiology during the early decades of the century, introduced the term *hormone* for the internal secretions of the endocrine glands. In 1891 the English physician George Redmayne Murray achieved the first success in treating myxedema (the common form of hypothyroidism) with an extract of the thyroid gland. Three years later, Sharpey-Schafer and George Oliver demonstrated in extracts of the adrenal glands a substance that raised the blood pressure; and in 1901 Jokichi Takamine, a Japanese chemist working in the United States, isolated this active principle, known as epinephrine or adrenaline.

EPINEPHRINE AND NOREPINEPHRINE

Epinephrine and norepinephrine, also known as adrenaline and noradrenaline, are two separate but related hormones that are secreted by the medulla of the adrenal glands. They are also produced at the ends of sympathetic nerve fibres, where they serve as chemical mediators for conveying the nerve impulses to effector organs. Chemically, the two compounds differ only slightly; and they exert similar pharmacological actions, which resemble the effects of stimulation of the sympathetic nervous system. They are, therefore, classified as sympathomimetic agents. The active secretion of the adrenal medulla contains approximately 80 percent epinephrine and 20 percent norepinephrine. But this proportion is reversed in the sympathetic nerves, which contain predominantly norepinephrine.

The actions of epinephrine and norepinephrine are generally similar, although they differ from each other in certain of their effects. Norepinephrine constricts almost all blood vessels, while epinephrine causes constriction in many networks of minute blood vessels but dilates the blood vessels in the skeletal muscles and the liver. Both hormones increase the rate and force of contraction of the heart, thus increasing the output of blood from the heart and increasing the blood pressure. The hormones also have important metabolic actions. Epinephrine stimulates the breakdown of glycogen to glucose in the liver, which results in the raising of the level of blood sugar. Both hormones increase the level of circulating free fatty acids. The extra amounts of glucose and fatty acids can be used by the body as fuel in times of stress or danger where increased alertness or exertion is required. Epinephrine is sometimes called the emergency hormone because it is released during stress and its stimulatory effects fortify and prepare an animal for either "fight or flight."

The purified, active compounds are used clinically and are obtained from the adrenal glands of domesticated animals or prepared synthetically. Epinephrine may be injected into the hearts of victims of cardiac arrest to stimulate heart activity. It also dilates the bronchioles and in this way is an aid to respiration for asthma sufferers. Epinephrine is also useful in acute allergic disorders, such as drug reactions, hives, and hay fever. Norepinephrine is administered by intravenous infusion to combat the acute fall in blood pressure associated with certain types of shock. Norepinephrine is formed in the body from the amino acid tyrosine, and epinephrine is in turn formed from norepinephrine. The Swedish physiologist Ulf von Euler discovered norepinephrine in the mid-1940s.

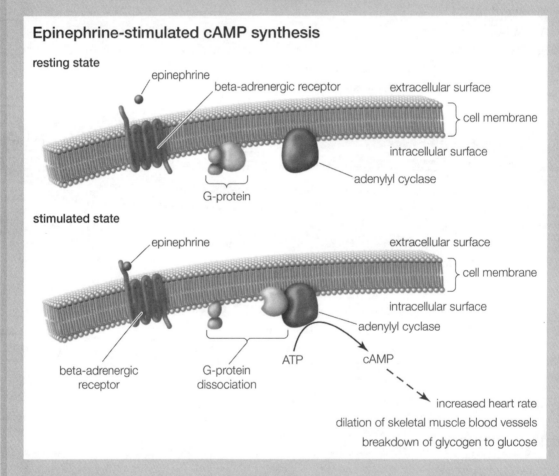

In cells the stimulatory effects of epinephrine are mediated through the activation of a second messenger known as cAMP (cyclic adenosine monophosphate). The activation of this molecule results in the stimulation of cell-signaling pathways that act to increase heart rate, to dilate blood vessels in skeletal muscle, and to break down glycogen to glucose in the liver. Encyclopædia Britannica, Inc.

INSULIN

During the first two decades of the 20th century, steady progress was made in the isolation, identification, and study of the active principles of the various endocrine glands, but the outstanding event of the early years was the discovery of insulin by Frederick Banting, Charles H. Best, and J.J.R. Macleod in 1921. Almost overnight the lot of the diabetic patient changed from a sentence of almost certain death to a prospect not only of survival but of a long and healthy life.

For more than 30 years, some of the greatest minds in physiology had been seeking the cause of diabetes mellitus. In 1889 the German physicians Joseph von Mering and Oskar Minkowski had shown that removal of the pancreas in dogs produced the disease. In 1901 the American pathologist Eugene L. Opie described degenerative changes in the clumps of cells in the pancreas known as the islets of Langerhans, thus confirming the association between failure in the function of these cells and diabetes. Sharpey-Schafer concluded that the islets of Langerhans secrete a substance that controls the metabolism of carbohydrate. Then Banting, Best, and Macleod, working at the University of Toronto, succeeded in isolating the elusive hormone and gave it the name insulin.

Insulin was available in a variety of forms, but synthesis on a commercial scale was not achieved, and the only source of the hormone was the pancreas of animals. One of its practical disadvantages is that it has to be given by injection. Consequently an intense search was conducted for some alternative substance that would be active when taken by mouth. Various preparations—oral hypoglycemic agents, as they are known—appeared that were effective to a certain extent in controlling diabetes, but evidence indicated that these were only of value in relatively mild cases of the disease. For the person with advanced diabetes, a normal, healthy life remained dependent upon the continuing use of insulin injections.

CORTISONE

Another major advance in endocrinology came from the Mayo Clinic, in Rochester, Minn. In 1949 Philip Showalter Hench and his colleagues announced that a substance isolated from the cortex of the adrenal gland had a dramatic effect upon rheumatoid arthritis. This was compound E, or cortisone, as it came to be known, which had been isolated by Edward C. Kendall in 1935. Cortisone and its many derivatives proved to be potent as anti-inflammatory agents. Although it is not a cure for rheumatoid arthritis, as a temporary measure cortisone can often control the acute exacerbation caused by the disease and can provide relief in other conditions, such as acute rheumatic fever, certain kidney diseases, certain serious diseases of the skin, and some allergic conditions, including acute exacerbations of asthma. Of even more long-term importance is the valuable role it has as a research tool.

SEX HORMONES

Not the least of the advances in endocrinology was the increasing knowledge and understanding of the sex hormones. This culminated in the application of this knowledge to the problem of birth control. After an initial stage of hesitancy, the contraceptive pill, with its basic rationale of preventing ovulation, was accepted by the vast majority of family-planning organizations and many gynecologists as the most satisfactory method of contraception. Its risks, practical and theoretical, introduced a note of caution, but this was not sufficient to detract from the wide appeal induced by its effectiveness and ease of use.

NUTRITION AND VITAMINS

In the field of nutrition, the outstanding advance of the 20th century was the discovery and the appreciation of the importance to health of the "accessory food factors," or vitamins. Various workers had shown that animals did not thrive on a synthetic diet containing all the correct amounts of protein, fat, and carbohydrate. They even suggested that there must be some unknown ingredients in natural food that were essential for growth and the maintenance of health. But little progress was made in this field until the classical experiments of the

English biologist F. Gowland Hopkins were published in 1912. These were so conclusive that there could be no doubt that what he termed "accessory substances" were essential for health and growth. The name *vitamine* was suggested for these substances by the biochemist Casimir Funk in the belief that they were amines, certain compounds derived from ammonia. In due course, when it was realized that they were not amines, the term was altered to *vitamin*.

Once the concept of vitamins was established on a firm scientific basis it was not long before their identity began to be revealed. Soon there was a long series of vitamins, best known by the letters of the alphabet after which they were originally named when their chemical identity was still unknown. By supplementing the diet with foods containing particular vitamins, deficiency diseases such as rickets (due to deficiency of vitamin D) and scurvy (due to lack of vitamin C, or ascorbic acid) practically disappeared from Western countries, while deficiency diseases such as beriberi (caused by lack of vitamin B1, or thiamine), which were endemic in Eastern countries, either disappeared or could be remedied with the greatest of ease.

The isolation of vitamin B12, or cyanocobalamin, was of particular interest because it almost rounded off the fascinating story of how pernicious anemia was brought under control. Throughout the first two decades of the century, the diagnosis of pernicious anemia, like that of diabetes mellitus, was nearly equivalent to a death sentence. Unlike the more common form of so-called secondary anemia, it did not respond to the administration of suitable iron salts, and no other form of treatment touched it. Hence, the grimly appropriate title of pernicious anemia.

In the early 1920s, George R. Minot, one of the many brilliant investigators that Harvard University has contributed to medical research, became interested in work being done by the American pathologist George H. Whipple on the beneficial effects of raw beef liver in severe experimental anemia. With a Harvard colleague, William P. Murphy, he decided to investigate the effect of raw liver in patients with pernicious anemia, and in 1926 they were able to announce that this form of therapy was successful. The validity of their findings was amply confirmed, and the fear of pernicious anemia came to an end.

As so often happens in medicine, many years were to pass before the rationale of liver therapy in pernicious anemia was fully understood. In 1948, however, almost simultaneously in the United States and Britain, the active principle, cyanocobalamin, was isolated from liver, and this vitamin became the standard treatment for pernicious anemia.

TROPICAL MEDICINE

The first half of the 20th century witnessed the virtual conquest of three of the major diseases of the tropics: malaria, yellow fever, and leprosy. At the turn of the century, as for the preceding two centuries, quinine was the only known drug to have any appreciable effect on malaria. With the increasing development of tropical countries and rising standards of public health, it became obvious that quinine was not completely satisfactory. Intensive research between World Wars I and II indicated that several synthetic compounds were more effective. The first of these to become available, in 1934, was quinacrine (known as mepacrine, Atabrine, or Atebrin). In World War II it amply fulfilled the highest expectations and helped to reduce disease among Allied troops in Africa, Southeast Asia, and the Far East. A number of other effective antimalarial drugs subsequently became available.

An even brighter prospect—the virtual eradication of malaria—was opened up by the introduction, during World War II, of the insecticide DDT (1,1,1-trichloro-2,2,-bis[p-chlorophenyl]ethane, or dichloro-diphenyltrichloro-ethane). It had long been realized that the only effective way of controlling malaria was to eradicate the anopheline mosquitoes that transmit the disease. Older methods of mosquito control, however, were cumbersome and expensive. The lethal effect of DDT on the mosquito, its relative cheapness, and its ease of use on a widespread scale provided the answer. An intensive worldwide campaign, sponsored by the World Health Organization, was planned and went far toward bringing malaria under control.

The major problem encountered with respect to effectiveness was that

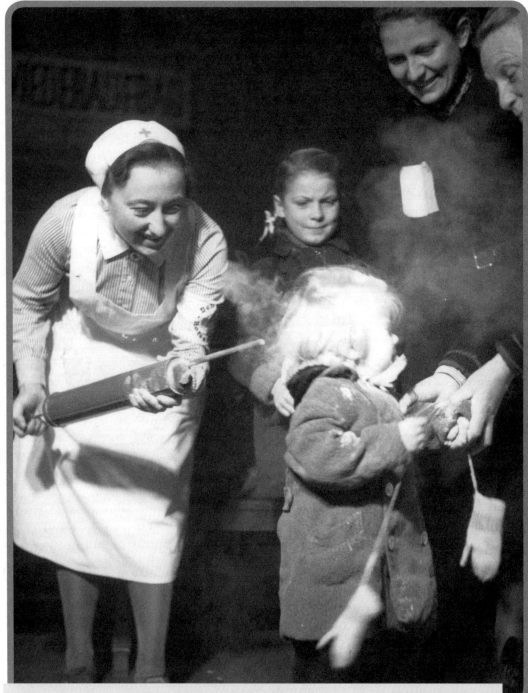

A child cries as she is sprayed with DDT delousing powder in Wilmerssdorf, Germany, in October 1945. George Konig/Hulton Archive/Getty Images

the mosquitoes were able to develop a resistance to DDT. But the introduction of other insecticides, such as dieldrin and lindane (BHC), helped to overcome this difficulty. The use of DDT, dieldrin, and other insecticides, however, was strongly criticized because of their devastating effects on the environment. Concerns that DDT endangered wildlife, the environment, and human health (concerns that stemmed mainly from the chemical's widespread use in agriculture) led to the banning of DDT in many countries, including the United States in 1972. In the 21st century, however, the World Health Organization (WHO), which had long supported the ban on DDT, reversed its position and recommended the use of the chemical as a principal tool in the ongoing war against malaria.

Yellow fever is another mosquito-transmitted disease, and the prophylactic value of modern insecticides in its control was almost as great as in the case of malaria. The forest reservoirs of the virus present a more difficult problem, but the combined use of immunization and insecticides did much to bring this disease under control.

Until the 1940s the only drugs available for treating leprosy were the chaulmoogra oils and their derivatives. These, though helpful, were far from satisfactory. In the 1940s the group of drugs known as the sulfones appeared, and it soon became apparent that they were infinitely better than any other group of drugs in the treatment of leprosy. Several other drugs later proved promising. In

the 21st century, a multidrug regimen developed by WHO provided an effective means by which leprosy could be managed. The three drugs used in WHO's regimen included dapsone, clofazimine, and rifampicin. The latter was also used in the treatment of tuberculosis.

NOTABLE FIGURES IN THE ADVANCEMENT OF 20TH-CENTURY MEDICINE

Underlying the progress in endocrinology and tropical medicine in the 20th century was the work of numerous physicians and researchers. The many and varied contributions of these individuals embody the era's ambitious attitude of discovery, and their breakthroughs in the areas of metabolism, nutrition, and infectious disease have had lasting impacts on the study and practice of medicine.

SIR FREDERICK BANTING
(b. Nov. 14, 1891, Alliston, Ont., Can.—d. Feb. 21, 1941, Newfoundland)

Canadian physician Sir Frederick Banting, with Charles H. Best, was the first to extract (1921) the hormone insulin from the pancreas. Injections of insulin proved to be the first effective treatment for diabetes, a disease in which glucose accumulates in abnormally high quantities in the blood. Banting was awarded a share of the 1923 Nobel Prize for Physiology or Medicine for his achievement.

Banting was educated at the University of Toronto, served in World War I, and then practiced medicine in London, Ont. In 1889 Joseph von Mering and Oskar Minkowski had found that complete removal of the pancreas in dogs immediately caused severe diabetes. Later scientists hypothesized that the pancreas controlled glucose metabolism by generating a hormone, which they named "insulin." However, repeated efforts to extract insulin from the pancreas ended in failure, because the pancreas' own digestive enzymes destroyed the insulin molecules as soon as the pancreas was ground up.

In May 1921 Banting and Charles Best, a medical student, began an intensive effort in the laboratories of the Scottish physiologist J.J.R. Macleod, at the University of Toronto, to isolate the hormone. By tying off the pancreatic ducts of dogs, they were able to reduce the pancreas to inactivity while preserving certain cells in the pancreas known as the islets of Langerhans, which were thought to be the site of insulin production. Solutions extracted from these cells were injected into the dogs whose pancreas had been removed, and the dogs quickly recovered from their artificially induced diabetes. Banting and Best were able to isolate insulin in a form that proved consistently effective in treating diabetes in humans. This discovery ultimately enabled millions of people suffering from diabetes to lead normal lives.

Banting and Best completed their experiments in 1922. The following year Banting and Macleod received the 1923 Nobel Prize for Physiology or Medicine for the discovery of insulin, though Macleod had not actually taken part in the original research. Angered that Macleod, rather than Best, had received the Nobel Prize, Banting divided his share of the award equally with Best. Macleod shared his portion of the Nobel Prize with James B. Collip, a young chemist who had helped with the purification of insulin. In 1923 Banting became head of the University of Toronto's Banting and Best Department of Medical Research. Banting was created a knight of the British Empire in 1934. He was killed in a plane crash in 1941 while on a war mission.

SIR WILLIAM MADDOCK BAYLISS
(b. May 2, 1860, Wolverhampton, Staffordshire, Eng.—d. Aug. 27, 1924, London)

British physiologist Sir William Maddock Bayliss was a codiscoverer (with the British physiologist Ernest Starling) of hormones. He also conducted pioneering research in major areas of physiology, biochemistry, and physical chemistry.

Bayliss studied at University College, London, and Wadham College, Oxford. He began a long and profitable collaboration with Starling soon after he obtained a teaching post at University College, London (1888), where he became professor of general physiology (1912–24). Their study in the 1890s of nerve-controlled contraction and dilation of blood vessels resulted in the development of an improved hemopiezometer (a device for measuring blood pressure). Observation of intestinal movements led to their discovery of the peristaltic wave, a rhythmic contraction that forces forward the contents of the intestine.

Bayliss and Starling are best known, however, for determining, in 1902, the chemical substance that stimulates the secretion of pancreatic digestive juices—the first example of hormonal action. In a famous experiment performed on anesthetized dogs, they showed that dilute hydrochloric acid, mixed with partially digested food, activates a chemical substance in the epithelial cells of the duodenum. They found that when this activated substance, which they called secretin, is released into the bloodstream, it comes into contact with the pancreas. There,it stimulates secretion of digestive juice into the intestine thorugh the pancreatic duct. They coined the term *hormone* (Greek *horman,* "to set in motion") to describe specific chemicals, such as secretin, that stimulate an organ at a distance from the chemical's site of origin. Bayliss went on to demonstrate how the enzyme trypsin was formed from inactive trypsinogen in the small intestine and to measure precisely the time required for a trypsin solution to digest specific quantities of protein.

Bayliss' World War I investigation of wound shock led him to recommend gum-saline injections that were responsible for saving many lives. He wrote *The Nature of Enzyme Action* (1908) and *The Vaso-Motor System* (1923). His best known work is *Principles of General Physiology* (1915), considered to be the best text on the subject at that time. He was knighted in 1922.

CHARLES H. BEST
(b. Feb. 27, 1899, West Pembroke, Maine, U.S.—d. March 31, 1978, Toronto, Ont., Can.)

American-born physiologist Charles H. Best, with Sir Frederick Banting, was the first to obtain (1921) a pancreatic extract of insulin in a form that controlled diabetes in dogs. The successful use of insulin in treating human patients followed. But because Best did not receive his medical degree until 1925, he did not share the Nobel Prize for Physiology or Medicine awarded to Banting and J.J.R. Macleod in 1923 for their role in the work. Best also discovered the vitamin choline and the enzyme histaminase. He was one of the first to introduce anticoagulants in treatment of thrombosis (blood clots).

In May 1921, while still an undergraduate, Best became a laboratory assistant to Banting at the University of Toronto. In the months that followed, they performed their prizewinning research on insulin. Best continued as research associate in the Banting and Best Department of Medical Research, which was created at the university in 1923, and he succeeded Banting as its director (1941–67). With Banting he wrote *Internal Secretions of the Pancreas* (1922).

ADOLF BUTENANDT
(b. March 24, 1903, Bremerhaven-Lehe, Ger.—d. Jan. 18, 1995, Munich)

German biochemist Adolf Butenandt, with Leopold Ružička, was awarded the 1939 Nobel Prize for Chemistry for his work on sex hormones. Although forced by the Nazi government to refuse the prize, he was able to accept the honour in 1949.

Butenandt studied at the universities of Marburg and Göttingen, receiving his Ph.D. from the latter in 1927. He then taught at Göttingen and at the Institute of Technology in Danzig (now Gdańsk, Pol.). Butenandt was director of the Kaiser Wilhelm Institute (later the Max Planck Institute) for Biochemistry in Berlin beginning in 1936, and when the institute moved to Tübingen in 1945 he became a professor at the University of Tübingen. In 1956, when the institute relocated to Munich, Butenandt became a professor at the University of Munich. He also served as president of the Max Planck Society for the Advancement of Science from 1960 to 1972.

In 1929, almost simultaneously with Edward A. Doisy in the United States, Butenandt isolated estrone, one of the hormones responsible for sexual development and function in females. In 1931 he isolated and identified androsterone, a male sex hormone, and in 1934, the hormone progesterone, which plays an important part in the female reproductive cycle. It was now clear that sex hormones are closely related to steroids, and after

Ružička showed that cholesterol could be transformed into androsterone, he and Butenandt were able to synthesize both progesterone and the male hormone testosterone. Butenandt's investigations made possible the eventual synthesis of cortisone and other steroids and led to the development of birth control pills.

In the 1940s Butenandt's researches on eye-colour defects in insects proved that specific genes control the synthesis of enzymes needed in various metabolic processes, and that mutations in those genes can result in metabolic defects. In 1959, after two decades of research, Butenandt and his colleagues isolated the sex attractant of the silkworm moth, *Bombyx mori*, which proved to be the first known example of the important class of chemical substances known as pheromones. He was also the first to crystallize an insect hormone, ecdysone.

CHRISTIAAN EIJKMAN
(b. Aug. 11, 1858, Nijkerk, Neth.—d. Nov. 5, 1930, Utrecht)

Dutch physician and pathologist Christiaan Eijkman demonstrated that beriberi is caused by poor diet. This realization led to the discovery of vitamins. Together with Sir Frederick Hopkins, he was awarded the 1929 Nobel Prize for Physiology or Medicine.

Eijkman received a medical degree from the University of Amsterdam (1883) and served as a medical officer in the Dutch East Indies (1883–85).

BERIBERI

Beriberi is a nutritional disorder caused by a deficiency of thiamin (vitamin B1). It is characterized primarily by impairment of the nerves and heart. General symptoms include loss of appetite and overall lassitude, digestive irregularities, and a feeling of numbness and weakness in the limbs and extremities. (The term beriberi *is derived from the Sinhalese word meaning "extreme weakness.") In the form known as dry beriberi, there is a gradual degeneration of the long nerves, first of the legs and then of the arms, with associated atrophy of muscle and loss of reflexes. In wet beriberi, a more acute form, there is edema (overabundance of fluid in the tissues) resulting largely from cardiac failure and poor circulation. In infants breast-fed by mothers who are deficient in thiamin, beriberi may lead to rapidly progressive heart failure.*

The cardiac symptoms, in both infants and adults, generally respond promptly and dramatically to the administration of thiamin. When neurological involvement is present, the response to thiamin is much more gradual. In severe cases, the structural lesions of the nerve cells may be irreversible. Thiamin normally plays an essential role as a coenzyme in the metabolism of carbohydrates. In its absence, pyruvic acid and lactic acid (products of carbohydrate digestion) accumulate in the tissues, where they are believed to be responsible for most of the neurological and cardiac manifestations.

Thiamin occurs widely in food but may be lost in the course of processing, particularly in the milling of grains. In East Asian countries, where polished white rice is a dietary staple, beriberi has been a long-standing problem. The history of the recognition, the cause, and the cure of beriberi is dramatic and is well documented in medical literature. In the 1880s the Japanese navy reported that beriberi had been eradicated among its sailors as a result of adding extra meat, fish, and vegetables to their regular diet. Before that time, almost half of the sailors were likely to develop beriberi, and many died of it. In 1897 Christiaan Eijkman, working in the Dutch East Indies (now Indonesia), found that a beriberi-like disease could be produced in chickens by feeding them a diet of polished rice. British researchers William Fletcher, Henry Fraser, and A.T. Stanton later confirmed that beriberi in humans was also related to the consumption of polished white rice. In 1912 Casimir Funk demonstrated that beriberi-like symptoms induced in pigeons could be cured by feeding them white rice that was supplemented with a concentrate made from rice polishings. Following this discovery he proposed that this, as well as several other conditions, were due to diets that were deficient in specific factors that he called "vitamines," later called vitamins.

The prevention of beriberi is accomplished by eating a well-balanced diet, since thiamin is present in most raw and untreated foods. The incidence of beriberi in Asia has markedly decreased because an improved standard of living has allowed a more varied diet and partly because of the gradual popular acceptance of partially dehusked, parboiled, and enriched rice—forms that contain higher concentrations of thiamin. In Western countries, thiamin deficiency is encountered almost solely in cases of chronic alcoholism.

He then worked with Robert Koch in Berlin on bacteriological research and in 1886 returned to Java to investigate the cause of beriberi. In 1888 Eijkman was appointed director of the research laboratory for pathological anatomy and bacteriology and of the Javanese Medical School in Batavia (now Jakarta). Eijkman sought a bacterial cause for beriberi. In 1890 polyneuritis broke out among his laboratory chickens. Noticing this disease's striking resemblance to the polyneuritis occurring in beriberi, he was eventually (1897) able to show that the condition was caused by feeding the fowl a diet of polished, rather than unpolished, rice.

Eijkman believed that the polyneuritis was caused by a toxic chemical agent, possibly originating from the action of intestinal microorganisms on boiled rice. He maintained this theory even after his successor in Batavia, Gerrit Grijns, demonstrated (1901) that the problem was a nutritional deficiency, later determined to be a lack of vitamin B1 (thiamine). Eijkman returned to the Netherlands in 1896 to serve as a professor at the University of Utrecht (1898–1928).

PHILIP SHOWALTER HENCH
(b. Feb. 28, 1896, Pittsburgh, Pa., U.S.—d. March 30, 1965, Ocho Rios, Jam.)

American physician Philip Showalter Hench, with Edward C. Kendall, in 1948 successfully applied an adrenal hormone (later known as cortisone) in the treatment of rheumatoid arthritis. With Kendall and

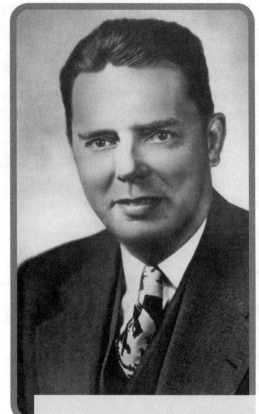

Philip Showalter Hench. Archiv für Kunst und Geschichte, Berlin

Tadeus Reichstein of Switzerland, Hench received the Nobel Prize for Physiology or Medicine in 1950 for discoveries concerning hormones of the adrenal cortex, their structure and biological effects.

Hench received his medical degree from the University of Pittsburgh in 1920 and spent almost his entire career at the Mayo Clinic in Rochester, Minn. For many years he sought a method of treating the painful and crippling disease of rheumatoid arthritis. Working at the Mayo Clinic, he noticed that during pregnancy and in the presence of jaundice the severe pain of arthritis may decrease and even disappear. This led him to suspect that arthritis is caused by a biochemical disturbance, perhaps one involving glandular hormones, rather than by a bacterial infection. In search of a treatment he and Kendall studied endocrinologic factors in rheumatic diseases. In the mid-1940s Kendall synthesized the steroid hormone cortisone, and in 1948 he and Hench tried the drug on arthritic patients. They showed a remarkable improvement, and cortisone became a key drug in the treatment of rheumatoid arthritis. Cortisone and similar steroids are still useful in treating a number of diseases, but the claims that greeted their early employment were excessive.

SIR FREDERICK GOWLAND HOPKINS
(b. June 20, 1861, Eastbourne, East Sussex, Eng.—d. May 16, 1947, Cambridge)

British biochemist Sir Frederick Gowland Hopkins received (with Christiaan Eijkman) the 1929 Nobel Prize for Physiology or Medicine for the discovery of nutrients needed in animal diets to maintain health.

Hopkins discovered the amino acid tryptophan in 1901, and he subsequently isolated it from protein. In 1906–07 he demonstrated that tryptophan and certain other amino acids (known as essential amino acids) cannot be manufactured by certain animals from other nutrients and must be supplied in the diet. He also showed that working muscles accumulate lactic acid. In 1922 he isolated the tripeptide glutathione and discovered its vital role in cellular oxygen metabolism. He was knighted in 1925 and received many other honours, including the presidency of the Royal Society (1930) and the Order of Merit (1935).

EDWARD CALVIN KENDALL
(b. March 8, 1886, South Norwalk, Conn., U.S.—d. May 4, 1972, Princeton, N.J.)

American chemist Edward Calvin Kendall, with Philip S. Hench and Tadeus Reichstein, won the Nobel Prize for Physiology or Medicine in 1950 for research on the structure and biological effects of adrenal cortex hormones.

A graduate of Columbia University (Ph.D. 1910), Kendall joined the staff of the Mayo Foundation, Rochester, Minn., in 1914. His early research concerned the isolation of the active constituent (thyroxine) of the thyroid hormone. He also crystallized and established the chemical nature of glutathione, a compound important to biological oxidation-reduction reactions.

Kendall's most important research, however was the isolation from the adrenal cortex of the steroid hormone cortisone (which he originally called compound E; 1935). With Hench, he successfully applied the hormone in treatment of rheumatoid arthritis (1948). Kendall and Hench, along with Reichstein of Switzerland, received a Nobel Prize in

1950, and Kendall retired from his position as head of the biochemistry division of the Mayo Foundation in 1951. Kendall also acted as head of the biochemistry laboratory there from 1945 to 1951, and he was later visiting professor of chemistry at Princeton University.

J.J.R. MACLEOD
(b. Sept. 6, 1876, Cluny, near Dunkeld, Perth, Scot.—d. March 16, 1935, Aberdeen)

Scottish physiologist J.J.R. Macleod was noted as a teacher and for his work on carbohydrate metabolism. Together with Sir Frederick Banting, with whom he shared the Nobel Prize for Physiology or Medicine in 1923, and Charles H. Best, he achieved renown as one of the discoverers of insulin.

Macleod held posts in physiology and biochemistry at the London Hospital (1899–1902) and as professor of physiology at Western Reserve University, Cleveland, Ohio, U.S. (1903–18). In 1918 he joined the University of Toronto, Ont., Can., as associate dean of medicine and subsequently became director of its physiological laboratory. It was in this laboratory that Banting and Best began investigating the secretions of the pancreas and eventually succeeded in isolating and preparing insulin in 1921. Macleod subsequently was made dean of the faculty of medicine. His publications include *Practical Physiology* (1902) and *Physiology and Biochemistry in Modern Medicine* (1918).

GEORGE RICHARDS MINOT
(b. Dec. 2, 1885, Boston, Mass., U.S.—d. Feb. 25, 1950, Brookline, Mass.)

American physician George Richards Minot received (with George H. Whipple and William P. Murphy) the Nobel Prize for Physiology or Medicine in 1934 for the introduction of a raw-liver diet in the treatment of pernicious anemia, which was previously an invariably fatal disease.

Minot received his medical degree at Harvard University in 1912. He did research at the Massachusetts General Hospital, Boston (1915–23), the Collis P. Huntington Memorial Hospital, Harvard University (1922–28), and the Peter Bent Brigham Hospital, Boston (1923–28). He served as director of the Thorndike Memorial Laboratory, Boston City Hospital, from 1928 until his death. Diagnosed with diabetes in 1921, his ability to work was hindered until he began using insulin in 1923, which had been synthesized for the first time the year before and is considered to have saved his life.

Whipple had shown that anemia in dogs, induced by excessive bleeding, is reversed by a diet of raw liver, and in 1926 he and Murphy found that ingestion of a half pound of raw liver a day dramatically reversed pernicious anemia in human beings. With the American chemist Edwin Cohn, Minot succeeded in preparing effective liver extracts, which, taken orally, constituted the primary treatment for pernicious anemia until 1948, when a therapeutic factor was isolated and named vitamin B12.

WILLIAM P. MURPHY
(b. Feb. 6, 1892, Stoughton, Wis., U.S.—d. Oct. 9, 1987, Brookline, Mass.)

American physician William P. Murphy, with George R. Minot, in 1926 reported success in the treatment of pernicious anemia with a liver diet. The two men shared the Nobel Prize for Physiology or Medicine in 1934 with George H. Whipple, whose research they had built upon.

Murphy received his M.D. from Harvard University (1920). He joined the staff of Peter Bent Brigham Hospital (later Brigham and Women's Hospital) in Boston in 1923, where he began his collaboration with Minot. Whipple in the early 1920s had demonstrated that liver in the diet sharply raised red blood cell counts in anemic patients. Acting on this cue, Minot, assisted by Murphy, began feeding liver to their pernicious anemia patients, with amazing results. Their discovery converted pernicious anemia from an often-fatal disease into a treatable disorder and laid the groundwork for the development in 1948 of vitamin B12 therapy. Murphy continued to serve at the Brigham Hospital and also taught at Harvard University from 1923. He retired in 1958. His textbook *Anemia in Practice* was published in 1939.

GEORGE REDMAYNE MURRAY
(b. June 20, 1865, Newcastle-upon-Tyne, Northumberland, Eng.—d. Sept. 21, 1939, Mobberley, Cheshire)

English physician George Redmayne Murray was a pioneer in the treatment of endocrine disorders. He was one of the first to use extractions of animal thyroid to relieve myxedema (severe hypothyroidism) in humans.

Murray, the son of a prominent physician, William Murray, received clinical training at University College Hospital, London. He was awarded both his M.B. (1889) and M.D. (1896) by the University of Cambridge. Determined to pursue a career in experimental medicine, Murray in 1891 became pathologist to the Hospital for Sick Children in Newcastle. He also lectured in bacteriology and comparative anatomy at Durham University. From 1893 to 1908 he was Heath professor of comparative pathology at Durham. Appointed to the chair of medicine at Manchester University, he remained there to the end of his career.

In 1891 Murray published his most important research, a report in the *British Medical Journal* on the effectiveness of sheep thyroid extract in treating myxedema in humans. Thyroid deficiency had been recognized as the cause of myxedema in the 1880s, and several researchers had established that an animal could survive the usually fatal effects of thyroidectomy if part of the excised thyroid gland was transplanted to another body location. Sir Victor Horsley, a colleague of Murray's, later suggested that part of a sheep's thyroid could be transplanted into human patients to relieve myxedema. Murray surmised, however, that a hypodermic injection of thyroid extract could more effectively be used to correct myxedema in humans, and he was completely successful in his first such attempt at treatment. Subsequent tests substantiated his approach.

TADEUS REICHSTEIN
(b. July 20, 1897, Włocławek, Pol.—d. Aug. 1, 1996, Basel, Switz.)

Swiss chemist Tadeus Reichstein, with Philip S. Hench and Edward C. Kendall, received the Nobel Prize for Physiology or Medicine in 1950 for his discoveries concerning hormones of the adrenal cortex.

Reichstein was educated in Zürich and held posts in the department of organic chemistry at the Federal Institute of Technology, Zürich, from 1930. From 1946 to 1967 he was professor of organic chemistry at the University of Basel. He received the Nobel Prize for research carried out independently on the steroid hormones produced by the adrenal cortex, the outer layer of the adrenal gland. Reichstein and his colleagues isolated about 29 hormones and determined their structure and chemical composition. One of the hormones they isolated, cortisone, was later discovered to be an anti-inflammatory agent useful in the treatment of arthritis. Reichstein was also involved in developing methods to synthesize the hormones he had discovered, among them cortisone and desoxycorticosterone, which was used for many years to treat Addison's disease.

Apart from hormone research, Reichstein is also known for his synthesis of vitamin C, a feat achieved about the same time (1933) in England by Sir Walter N. Haworth and coworkers. In the latter part of his career, Reichstein studied plant glycosides, chemicals that can be used in the development of therapeutic drugs. He was awarded the Copley Medal of the British Royal Society in 1968.

LEOPOLD RUŽIČKA
(b. Sept. 13, 1887, Vukovar, Croatia, Austria-Hungary [now in Croatia]—d. Sept. 26, 1976, Zürich, Switz.)

Swiss chemist Leopold Ružička was a joint recipient, with Adolf Butenandt of Germany, of the 1939 Nobel Prize for Chemistry for his work on ringed molecules, terpenes (a class of hydrocarbons found in the essential oils of many plants), and sex hormones.

While working as an assistant to the German chemist Hermann Staudinger, Ružička investigated the composition of the insecticides in pyrethrum (1911–16). Accompanying Staudinger to the Federal Institute of Technology in Zürich, he became a Swiss citizen and lectured at the institute. In 1926 he became professor of organic chemistry at the University of Utrecht in the Netherlands, and three years later he returned to Switzerland to become professor of chemistry at the Federal Institute of Technology.

Ružička's investigations of natural odoriferous compounds, begun in 1916, culminated in the discovery that the molecules of muskone and civetone, important to the perfume industry, contain rings of 15 and 17 carbon atoms, respectively. Before this discovery, rings with more than eight atoms had been unknown and indeed had been believed to be too unstable to exist. Ružička's discovery greatly expanded research on these compounds. He also showed that the carbon skeletons of terpenes and many other large organic molecules are constructed from multiple units of isoprene. In the mid-1930s Ružička discovered the molecular structure of several male sex hormones, notably testosterone and androsterone, and subsequently synthesized them.

ERNEST HENRY STARLING
(b. April 17, 1866, London, Eng.—d. May 2, 1927, Kingston Harbour, Jamaica)

British physiologist Ernest Henry Starling was known for his prolific contributions to a modern understanding of body functions, especially the maintenance of a fluid balance throughout the tissues, the regulatory role of endocrine secretions, and mechanical controls on heart function. These discoveries made him one of the foremost scientists of his time.

While serving as an instructor (1889–99) at Guy's Hospital, London M.D., 1890, Starling undertook investigations of lymph secretion that resulted in his clarification of the nature of fluid exchanges between vessels and tissues. Formulating what is known as Starling's

hypothesis (1896), he stated that, because the capillary wall may be considered a semipermeable membrane, allowing salt solutions to pass freely through it, the hydrostatic pressure forcing these solutions into tissues is balanced by the osmotic pressure—generated by colloidal (protein) solutions trapped in the capillary—forcing an absorption of fluid from the tissues.

As professor of physiology at University College, London (1899–1923), Starling began a highly profitable collaboration with the British physiologist William Bayliss that immediately saw their demonstration (1899) of the nervous control of the peristaltic wave, the muscle action responsible for the movement of food through the intestine. In 1902 they isolated a substance that they called secretin, released into the blood from the epithelial cells of the duodenum (between the stomach and small intestine), which in turn stimulates secretion into the intestine of pancreatic digestive juice. Two years later, Starling coined the term *hormone* to denote such substances released in a restricted part of the body (endocrine gland), carried by the bloodstream to unconnected parts, where, in extremely small quantities, they are capable of profoundly influencing the function of those parts.

After government-sponsored World War I research concerning poison gas defense, Starling developed an isolated heart-lung preparation that enabled him to formulate (1918) his "law of the heart," stating that the force of muscular contraction of the heart is directly proportional to the extent to which the muscle is stretched. Studying kidney function, he found (1924) that water, chlorides, bicarbonates, and glucose, lost in the excretory filtrate, are reabsorbed at the lower end of the kidney tubules (glomeruli). His *Principles of Human Physiology* (1912), continually revised, was a standard international text.

JOKICHI TAKAMINE
(b. Nov. 3, 1854, Takaoka, Japan—d. July 22, 1922, New York, N.Y., U.S.)

Japanese-born biochemist and industrial leader Jokichi Takamine isolated the chemical adrenalin (now called epinephrine) from the suprarenal gland (1901). This was the first pure hormone to be isolated from natural sources.

The son of a physician, Takamine graduated (1879) as a chemical engineer from the College of Science and Engineering of the Imperial University of Tokyo. The Japanese government sent him to Glasgow for postgraduate study at the university and at Anderson's College. During vacations he visited industrial plants, observing the manufacture of soda and fertilizers. After his return to Japan, Takamine entered the Imperial Department of Agriculture and Commerce; he rose rapidly, becoming head of the department's chemistry division. His first visit to the United States

was in 1884 as a commissioner to the Cotton Centennial Exposition in New Orleans. In 1887 Takamine left government service in order to establish his own factory, the Tokyo Artificial Fertilizer Co., which manufactured superphosphate fertilizers.

In his private laboratory, Takamine developed, from a fungus grown on rice, a starch-digesting enzyme similar to diastase. He named this new enzyme Takadiastase. In 1890 he was called to the United States to devise a practical application of the enzyme for the distilling industry. At this time he took up permanent residence in the United States, establishing the laboratory at Clifton, N.J., where his pioneering research in the isolation of adrenalin was carried out. The production of Takadiastase for medicinal use was taken over by the Parke-Davis Co., with whom Takamine was associated for the remainder of his career. He maintained close ties with Japan, aiding its development of industrial dyes, aluminum fabrication, nitrogen fixation, the electric furnace, and the manufacture of Bakelite.

GEORGE H. WHIPPLE
(b. Aug. 28, 1878, Ashland, N.H., U.S.—d. Feb. 1, 1976, Rochester, N.Y.),

American pathologist George H. Whipple discovered that raw liver fed to chronically bled dogs can reverse the effects of anemia. His findings led directly to successful liver treatment of pernicious anemia by the American physicians George R. Minot and William P. Murphy. This major advance in the treatment of noninfectious diseases brought the three men the Nobel Prize for Physiology or Medicine in 1934.

After obtaining a medical degree from Johns Hopkins University (Baltimore) in 1905, Whipple began in 1908 a study of bile pigments. This led to his interest in the body's manufacture of the oxygen-carrying hemoglobin, which is also an important constituent in the production of bile pigments. In 1920 he demonstrated that liver as a dietary factor greatly enhances hemoglobin regeneration in dogs. He also carried out experiments in artificial anemia (1923–25), which established iron as the most potent inorganic factor involved in the formation of red blood cells. Whipple worked at Johns Hopkins University and then the University of California, San Francisco, before moving to the University of Rochester, where he spent most of his career (1921–55) and was first dean of the School of Medicine and Dentistry.

CHAPTER 6

DEVELOPMENTS IN THE UNDERSTANDING OF CANCER

While progress was the hallmark of medicine after the beginning of the 20th century, there is one field in which a gloomier picture must be painted, that of malignant disease, or cancer. Cancer was the second most common cause of death in most Western countries in the second half of the 20th century, being exceeded only by deaths from heart disease. By the end of the century, however, substantial progress in the understanding, diagnosis, and treatment of cancer had been achieved. Although the causes of the various types of malignancies were not completely known, many more methods became available for attacking the problem. Surgery remained the principal therapeutic standby, but radiotherapy and chemotherapy were increasingly used.

ACHIEVING A BASIC UNDERSTANDING OF CANCER

Soon after the discovery of radium was announced, in 1898, its potentialities in treating cancer were realized. In due course it assumed an important role in therapy. Simultaneously, deep X-ray therapy was developed, and with the atomic age came the use of radioactive isotopes. (A radioactive isotope is an unstable variant of a substance that has a stable form; during the process of breaking down, the unstable form emits radiation.) High-voltage X-ray therapy and radioactive isotopes have largely replaced radium. Whereas irradiation long depended upon X rays generated at 250 kilovolts, machines that were capable of producing X rays generated at 8,000 kilovolts and betatrons of up to 22,000,000 electron volts (MeV) came into clinical use. The most effective of the isotopes was radioactive cobalt. Telecobalt machines (those that hold the cobalt at a distance from the body) were available containing 2,000 curies or more of the isotope, an amount equivalent to 3,000 grams of radium and sending out a beam equivalent to that from a 3,000-kilovolt X-ray machine.

Of even more significance were the developments in the chemotherapy of cancer. Nothing remotely resembling a chemotherapeutic cure has been achieved, but in certain forms of malignant disease, such as leukemia, which cannot be treated by surgery, palliative effects were achieved that prolong life and allow the patient in many instances to lead a comparatively normal existence.

Fundamentally, however, perhaps the most important advance of all in this field was the increasing appreciation of the importance of prevention. The discovery of the relationship between cigarette smoking and lung cancer is the classic example. Less publicized, but of equal import, was the continuing supervision of new techniques in industry and food manufacture in an attempt to ensure that they do not involve the use of cancer-causing substances.

Radium

Radium is a radioactive chemical element, the heaviest of the alkaline-earth metals of main Group 2 (IIa) of the periodic table. Radium is a silvery white metal that does not occur free in nature. It was discovered (1898) by Pierre Curie, Marie Curie, and an assistant, G. Bémont, after Marie Curie had observed that the radioactivity of pitchblende was four or five times greater than that of the uranium it contained and not fully explained on the basis of radioactive polonium, which she had just discovered in pitchblende residues. The new, powerfully radioactive substance could be concentrated with barium, but because its chloride was slightly more insoluble it could be concentrated by fractional crystallization. The separation was followed by the increase in intensity of new lines in the ultraviolet spectrum and by a steady increase in the apparent atomic weight of the material until a value of 225.18 was obtained, remarkably close to the accepted value of 226.03. By 1902, 0.1 gram of pure radium chloride was prepared by refining several tons of pitchblende residues, and by 1910 Marie Curie and André-Louis Debierne had isolated the metal itself.

Thirty-three isotopes of radium, all radioactive, are known. Their half-lives, except for radium-226 (1,600 years) and radium-228 (5.8 years), are less than a few weeks. The long-lived radium-226 is found in nature as a result of its continuous formation from uranium-238 decay. Radium thus occurs in all uranium ores, but it is more widely distributed because it forms water-soluble compounds. Earth's surface contains an estimated 1.8×10^{13} grams of radium.

Radium's uses all result from its radiations. The most important use of radium was formerly in medicine, principally for the treatment of cancer by subjecting tumours to the gamma radiation of its daughter isotopes. In many therapeutic applications radium has been superseded by the less costly and more powerful artificial radioisotopes cobalt-60 and cesium-137. An intimate mixture of radium and beryllium is a moderately intense source of neutrons, used for scientific research and for well logging in geophysical prospecting for petroleum. For these uses, however, substitutes have become available. One of the products of radium decay is radon, the heaviest noble gas. This decay process is the chief source of that element.

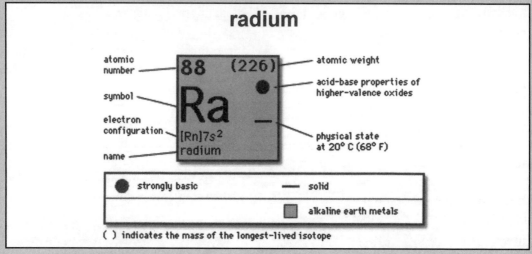

© 1997 Encyclopædia Britannica, Inc.

THE ROLE OF RETROVIRUSES

For many years there existed a paradigm in molecular biology known as the "central dogma." This asserted that DNA is first transcribed into RNA, RNA is translated into amino acids, and amino acids assemble into long chains, called polypeptides, that make up proteins—the functional units of cellular life. However, while this central dogma is true, as with many paradigms of biology, important exceptions can be found.

The first important observation opposing the central dogma came in the early 20th century. Two Danish researchers, Vilhelm Ellerman and Oluf Bang, were able to transmit leukemia to six chickens in succession by infecting the first animal with a filterable agent (now known as a virus) and then infecting each subsequent animal with the blood of the preceding bird. At the time, only palpable malignant tumours were understood to be cancers. Therefore, this observation was not linked to a viral-induced malignancy because leukemia was not then known to be a cancer. (At the time, leukemia was thought to be the result of some manner of bacterial infection.)

In 1911 American pathologist Peyton Rous, working at the Rockefeller Institute for Medical Research (now Rockefeller University), reported that healthy chickens developed malignant sarcomas (cancers of connective tissues) when infected with tumour cells from other chickens. Rous investigated the tumour cells further, and from them, he isolated a virus, which was later named Rous sarcoma virus (RSV). However, the concept of infectious cancer drew little support, and, unable to isolate viruses from other cancers, Rous abandoned the work in 1915 and did not return to it until 1934. Decades later the significance of his discoveries was realized, and in 1966—more than 55 years after his first experiment, at the age of 87—Rous was awarded the Nobel Prize for Physiology or Medicine for his discovery of tumour-inducing viruses.

In the mid-20th century there were many advances in molecular biology, including the description of DNA in 1953 by American geneticist and biophysicist James D. Watson and British biophysicists Francis Crick and Maurice Wilkins. By the 1960s it was understood that sarcomas are caused by a mutation that results in uncontrolled cell division. It was also evident that RSV was inherited during the division of cancerous cells. This inheritance occurred in a manner agreeing with the Mendelian laws of genetic inheritance—laws that heretofore had been understood to apply only to DNA molecules.

Scientists hypothesized that, in order for such viral inheritance to occur, a virus would need to transcribe its RNA genome into DNA and then insert this DNA into the host cell genome. Once incorporated into the host genome, the virus would be transcribed as though it were another gene and could produce more RNA virus from its DNA. This hypothesis, called the "DNA provirus hypothesis," was developed in the late 1950s by American virologist Howard Martin Temin, when he was a postdoctoral fellow in the laboratory of Italian virologist Renato Dulbecco at the California Institute of Technology. Temin's hypothesis was formally proposed in 1964. The provirus hypothesis came about when experiments demonstrated that an antibiotic called actinomycin D, which is capable of inhibiting DNA and RNA synthesis, inhibited the reproduction of RSV. However, the concept of an RNA molecule's turning itself into DNA drew very few supporters.

In 1970 Temin and Japanese virologist Satoshi Mizutani, and American virologist David Baltimore, working independently, reported the discovery of an enzyme that could synthesize proviral DNA from the RNA genome of RSV. This enzyme was named RNA-directed DNA polymerase, commonly referred to as reverse transcriptase. This discovery resulted in the identification of a unique virus family (Retroviridae), and the understanding of the pathogenesis of these viruses spurred a rush to discover other infectious cancer-causing agents.

In the early 1980s the HTLV-I and HTLV-II retroviruses were discovered and found to cause leukemia. In 1983 HIV (human immunodeficiency virus) was isolated and identified as the causative agent of AIDS. HIV infects white blood cells known as helper T cells and results in the production of more virus and, eventually, cell death and destruction of the immune system. In 2007 approximately 2.1 million people worldwide died of AIDS, an estimated 33.2 million people were living with HIV, and approximately 2.5 million people were newly infected with HIV. Drugs that inhibit reverse transcriptase were the first treatments available to people living with HIV. Nucleoside reverse transcriptase inhibitors (NRTIs) such as AZT (zidovudine)—the first drug approved by the U.S. Food and Drug Administration to prolong the lives of AIDS patients—act by terminating the proviral DNA chain before the enzyme can finish transcription. NRTIs are often given in combination with non-nucleoside reverse transcriptase inhibitors (NNRTIs) such as efavirenz that act by binding to and altering the shape of the enzyme itself, thereby blocking the enzyme's function.

The ability of reverse transcriptase to synthesize DNA from RNA has been used in the laboratory. For example, RT-PCR is commonly used to quantify the amount of messenger RNA (mRNA) transcribed from a gene. Because RNA is fragile and difficult to study, a strand of complementary DNA (cDNA) is synthesized from RNA, using reverse transcriptase during the RT-PCR procedure. The cDNA can then be amplified by polymerase chain reaction and used for subsequent experiments.

SMOKING AND HEALTH

The abundant use of tobacco products in the 20th century raised significant concerns about adverse health effects. Because tobacco was long considered to possess medicinal properties, however, shifts in medical and public perspectives were slow in coming. After decades of research, the link between smoking and lung cancer was firmly established in the latter part of the 20th century, and as a result, with much more known about the increased risk for lung and oral cancers, public attitudes reversed swiftly. No longer was tobacco advocated for relief of boredom or for enhancing mood. Rather, by the first decade of the 21st century, smoking bans had already been instituted in public areas in some cities and countries.

Smokers' tendency toward addiction to tobacco was realized in the 20th century. Thus, the rapid increase in smoking that occurred throughout the century raised significant concern that the incidence of smoking-related diseases and deaths would rise sharply in the 21st century. In the 1990s the World Health Organization (WHO) estimated that 4 million people died from tobacco-related disease annually. By 2003, this estimate was increased to 5 million. Based on the then current rate of tobacco consumption globally, experts further projected that by the start of the third decade of the 21st century, some 10 million people would die each year from tobacco smoking.

Most deaths from smoking cigarettes represent premature deaths, many of which are associated with the particulate matter from tobacco smoke, which increases the risk of cancer.

Indeed, more than 30 percent of all cancer deaths worldwide are attributable to tobacco. This is because, in addition to nicotine, tobacco products are often manufactured with various additives, which help to preserve shelf life and to make the product's flavours and aromas more appealing. However, studies have shown that tobacco smoke from products containing such additives contains around 4,000 chemical substances, the majority of which are toxic.

In fact, more than 60 known carcinogens (cancer-causing substances) are found in tobacco smoke. Examples of tobacco carcinogens include nitrosamines and polycyclic aromatic hydrocarbons. Cancer risk as a result of tobacco smoking is a function of exposure to carcinogens, particularly the amount and length of time of exposure. Hence, frequent smoking and smoking over the course of years increase the risk of developing a tobacco-related cancer substantially.

Carcinogens can bind to cellular DNA and cause genetic damage. Affected cells tend to then replicate uncontrollably, thereby giving rise to tumours, which become malignant, resulting in cancer. Cancer cells then spread to other parts of the body in a process known as metastasis. Once metastasis has occurred, a cancer may become impossible to treat.

In the United States lung cancer has become one of the most prevalent forms of cancer in both men and women. Some 85 percent of lung cancer cases are believed to be preventable. Thus, public health efforts focused on discouraging smoking have become paramount to reducing the loss of life from preventable disease.

MAJOR FIGURES IN THE HISTORY OF CANCER RESEARCH

Cancer as a disease was recognized long ago in the history of medicine. The Edwin Smith papyrus, an ancient Egyptian medical treatise dated to around 1600 BCE but believed to be a copy of a work dating from c. 3000 BCE, and the Ebers papyrus, an Egyptian compilation of medical texts dated to about 1550 BCE, contain some of the first written descriptions of tumours. In the 2nd century BCE the Greek physician Galen contemplated the causes of cancer and proposed surgical approaches for the treatment of advanced disease. A more complete understanding of cancer, however, did not emerge until the work of the physicians and scientists of the 18th, 19th, and 20th centuries became known. The contributions of individuals such as Sir Percivall Pott, who was the first to establish a link between cancer and environmental exposure, and David Baltimore, who contributed to the discovery of the role of retroviruses in cancer, were fundamental in providing the framework necessary for advancing cancer research into the 21st century.

David Baltimore
(b. March 7, 1938, New York, N.Y., U.S.)

American virologist David Baltimore shared the Nobel Prize for Physiology or Medicine in 1975 with Howard M. Temin and Renato Dulbecco. Working independently, Baltimore and Temin discovered reverse transcriptase, an enzyme that synthesizes DNA from RNA. Baltimore also conducted research that led to an understanding of the interaction between viruses and the genetic material of the cell. The research of all three men contributed to an understanding of the role of viruses in the development of cancer.

Baltimore and Temin both studied the process by which certain tumour-causing RNA viruses (those whose genetic material is composed of RNA) replicate after they infect a cell. They simultaneously demonstrated that these RNA viruses, now called retroviruses, contain the blueprint for an unusual enzyme—a polymerase called reverse transcriptase—that copies DNA from an RNA template. The newly formed viral DNA then integrates into the infected host cell, an event that can transform the infected cell into a cancer cell.

Baltimore received his undergraduate degree in chemistry from Swarthmore College, Pennsylvania (B.A., 1960), and went on to study animal virology at the Rockefeller Institute (now Rockefeller University) in New York City, where he obtained his doctorate in 1964, and at the Massachusetts Institute of Technology (MIT) in Boston. He worked with Dulbecco at the Salk Institute in La Jolla, California (1965–68), studying the mechanism of replication of the poliovirus.

Baltimore joined the faculty of MIT in 1968, accompanied by Alice Huang, a postdoctoral fellow who had worked on vesicular stomatitus virus (VSV) at the Salk Institute. In Boston, Baltimore and Huang, who had married, showed that VSV, an RNA virus, reproduced itself by means of an unusual enzyme (an RNA-dependent RNA polymerase) that copies RNA by a process not involving DNA.

Baltimore then turned his attention to two RNA tumour viruses—Rauscher murine leukemia virus and Rous sarcoma virus—to discover whether a similar enzyme was at work in their replication. It was through these experiments that he discovered reverse transcriptase. This discovery proved an exception to the "central dogma" of genetic theory, which states that the information encoded in genes always flows unidirectionally from DNA to RNA (and thence to proteins) and cannot be reversed. Since its discovery, reverse transcriptase has become an invaluable tool in recombinant DNA technology.

Baltimore became director of the Whitehead Institute for Biomedical Research in Cambridge, Massachusetts, in 1983 and in 1990 left to become president of Rockefeller University. In 1989 he figured prominently in a public dispute over a 1986 paper published in the journal *Cell* that he had coauthored while still at MIT. The coauthor of the article, Thereza Imanishi-Kari, was accused of falsifying data published in the paper.

Baltimore, who was not included in charges of misconduct, stood behind Imanishi-Kari, although he did retract the article. Because of his involvement in the case, however, he was asked to resign as president of Rockefeller University, and in 1994 he returned to MIT. In 1996 a U.S. government panel cleared Imanishi-Kari of the charges of scientific misconduct. The case was analyzed in *The Baltimore Case* (1998) by Daniel Kevles. Baltimore was president of the California Institute of Technology from 1997 to 2006, when he was elected to a three-year term as president of the American Association for the Advancement of Science (AAAS).

J. MICHAEL BISHOP
(b. Feb. 22, 1936, York, Pa., U.S.)

American virologist J. Michael Bishop was known for his achievements in clarifying the origins of cancer. He was awarded (with Harold Varmus) the 1989 Nobel Prize for Physiology or Medicine for his discoveries.

Bishop graduated from Gettysburg College (Pa.) in 1957 and from Harvard Medical School in 1962. After spending two years in internship and residency at Massachusetts General Hospital, Boston, he became a researcher in virology at the National Institutes of Health, Bethesda, Md. In 1968 he joined the faculty of the University of California Medical Center in San Francisco, becoming a full professor in 1972. From 1981 he also served as director of the university's George F. Hooper Research Foundation. In 1998

Bishop was elected chancellor of the University of California, San Francisco.

In 1970 Bishop teamed up with Varmus, and they set out to test the theory that healthy body cells contain dormant viral oncogenes that, when triggered, cause cancer. Working with the Rous sarcoma virus, known to cause cancer in chickens, Bishop and Varmus found that a gene similar to the cancer-causing gene within the virus was also present in healthy cells.

In 1976 Bishop and Varmus, together with two colleagues—Dominique Stehelin and Peter Vogt—published their findings, concluding that the virus had taken up the gene responsible for the cancer from a normal cell. After the virus had infected the cell and begun its usual process of replication, it incorporated the gene into its own genetic material. Subsequent research showed that such genes can cause cancer in several ways. Even without viral involvement, these genes can be converted by certain chemical carcinogens into a form that allows uncontrolled cellular growth.

Because the mechanism described by Bishop and Varmus seemed common to all forms of cancer, their work proved invaluable to cancer research. Today, scientists suspect that nearly 1 percent of the human genome, which contains approximately 25,000 genes, is made up of proto-oncogenes—genes that when altered or mutated from their original form have the ability to cause cancer in animals.

Bishop was awarded the National Medal of Science in 2003. That same year, he published *How to Win the Nobel Prize: An Unexpected Life in Science*, a reflection on his life and work that also touches on historical aspects of science and on the intellectual environment of modern-day research.

JOHANNES FIBIGER
(b. April 23, 1867, Silkeborg, Den.—d. Jan. 30, 1928, Copenhagen)

Danish pathologist Johannes Fibiger received the Nobel Prize for Physiology or Medicine in 1926 for achieving the first controlled induction of cancer in laboratory animals, a development of profound importance to cancer research.

A student of the bacteriologists Robert Koch and Emil von Behring in Berlin, Fibiger became professor of pathological anatomy at the University of Copenhagen (1900). In 1907, while dissecting rats infected with tuberculosis, he found tumours in the stomachs of three animals. After intensive research, he concluded that the tumours, apparently malignant, followed an inflammation of stomach tissue caused by the larvae of a worm now known as *Gongylonema neoplasticum*. The worms had infected cockroaches eaten by the rats.

By 1913 he was able to induce gastric tumours consistently in mice and rats by feeding them cockroaches infected with the worm. By showing that the tumours underwent metastasis, he added important support to the then-prevailing concept that cancer is caused by tissue irritation. Fibiger's work immediately led the Japanese pathologist Yamagiwa Katsusaburo to produce cancer in laboratory animals by painting their skins with coal-tar derivatives, a procedure soon adopted by Fibiger himself. While later research revealed that the *Gongylonema* larvae were not directly responsible for the inflammation, Fibiger's findings were a necessary prelude to the production of chemical carcinogens, a vital step in the development of modern cancer research.

CHARLES B. HUGGINS
(b. Sept. 22, 1901, Halifax, Nova Scotia, Can.—d. Jan. 12, 1997, Chicago, Ill., U.S.)

Canadian-born American surgeon and urologist Charles B. Huggins was noted for his investigations that demonstrated the relationship between hormones and certain types of cancer. For his discoveries Huggins received (with Peyton Rous) the Nobel Prize for Physiology or Medicine in 1966.

Huggins was educated at Acadia University (Wolfville, N.S.) and at Harvard University, where he received his M.D. in 1924. He went to the University of Michigan for further training in surgery (1924–27) and then joined the faculty of the University of Chicago, where he served as director of the Ben May Laboratory for Cancer Research from 1951 to 1969.

Huggins was a specialist on the male urological and genital tract. In the early 1940s he found he could retard the growth of prostate cancer by blocking the action of the patient's male hormones with doses of the female hormone estrogen. This research demonstrated that some cancer cells, like normal body cells, are dependent on hormonal signals to survive and grow and that, by depriving cancer cells of the correct signals, the growth of tumours could be slowed down, at least temporarily. In 1951 Huggins showed that breast cancers are also dependent on specific hormones. By removing the ovaries and adrenal glands, which are the source of estrogen, he could achieve significant tumour regression in some of his patients. Owing to his work, drugs that block the body's production of estrogen became important resources in treating breast cancer.

SALVADOR LURIA
(b. Aug. 13, 1912, Turin, Italy—d. Feb. 6, 1991, Lexington, Mass., U.S.)

Italian-born American biologist Salvador Luria (with Max Delbrück and Alfred Day Hershey) won the Nobel Prize for Physiology or Medicine in 1969 for research on bacteriophages, viruses that infect bacteria.

Luria graduated from the University of Turin in 1935 and became a radiology specialist. He fled Italy for France in 1938 and went to the United States in 1940 after learning the techniques of phage research at the Pasteur Institute in Paris. Soon after his arrival, he met Delbrück, through whom he became involved with the American Phage Group, an informal scientific organization devoted to solving the problems of viral self-replication. Working with a member of the group in

1942, Luria obtained one of the electron micrographs of phage particles, which confirmed earlier descriptions of them as consisting of a round head and a thin tail.

In 1943 Luria and Delbrück published a paper showing that, contrary to the current view, viruses undergo permanent changes in their hereditary material. That same year he and Delbrück devised the fluctuation test, which provided experimental evidence that phage-resistant bacteria were the result of spontaneous mutations rather than a direct response to changes in the environment. In 1945 Hershey and Luria demonstrated the existence not only of such bacterial mutants but also of spontaneous phage mutants.

Luria became Sedgwick professor of biology at the Massachusetts Institute of Technology in 1964. In 1974 he became director of the Center for Cancer Research at MIT. He was an author of a college textbook, *General Virology* (1953), and a popular text for the general reader, *Life: The Unfinished Experiment* (1973).

SIR PERCIVALL POTT
(b. Jan. 6, 1714, London, Eng.—d. Dec. 22, 1788, London)

English surgeon Sir Percivall Pott was noted for his many insightful and comprehensive surgical writings and was the first to associate cancer with occupational exposure.

Pott, whose father died when he was a young boy, was raised under the care of his mother and a relative, Joseph Wilcocks, the bishop of Rochester. He was sent to a private school in Kent and later was an apprentice to Edward Nourse, a surgeon at St. Bartholomew's Hospital in London. In preparing and dissecting cadavers for Nourse's anatomy classes, Pott not only became educated in the basic principles of anatomy and medicine but also eventually perfected his surgical technique. In 1736, after seven years under Nourse's instruction, Pott passed examinations for admittance to the Company of Barber Surgeons—the forerunner of the Royal College of Surgeons of England. The Company awarded Pott the Grand Diploma, an honorary achievement, in recognition for his exceptional surgical skills. In 1745 he became an assistant surgeon at St. Bartholomew's and was promoted to full surgeon in 1749.

In 1756, while on his way to see a patient, Pott was thrown from his horse and sustained an open compound fracture of his lower leg. He refused to allow his rescuers to move him right away. Instead, he instructed them to build a makeshift stretcher from a door and poles, which was used to carry him home. Several of his surgical colleagues examined the injury and recommended amputation, the standard course of treatment at the time. Nourse, however, who also went to see Pott, advised otherwise, suggesting reduction, in which traction and pressure are applied to the fracture to correct the positioning of the bones. Nourse's technique worked, and Pott's leg healed without complication. The reduction approach introduced by

Nourse was subsequently refined and became widely used in the treatment of open compound fracture, leading to a substantial decline in amputations. In addition, fractures of the lower leg similar to the type Pott suffered became known as Pott fracture. During his recovery, Pott wrote *A Treatise on Ruptures* (1756), a medical work in which he disproved misguided theories on the causes and treatment of hernias.

In *Chirurgical Observations Relative to the Cataract, the Polyplus of the Nose, the Cancer of the Scrotum, the Different Kinds of Ruptures, and the Mortification of the Toes and Feet* (1775), Pott published the first report of cancer caused by occupational exposure. He observed an unusually high incidence of skin sores on the scrotums of men working as chimney sweeps in London. He also discovered coal soot in the sores and eventually concluded that men routinely exposed to soot were at a high risk for scrotal cancer. Pott's report was the first in which an environmental factor was identified as a cancer-causing agent. The disease became known as chimney-sweepers' cancer, and Pott's work laid the foundation for occupational medicine and measures to prevent work-related disease.

Pott also described a disease of the vertebrae in which the bones soften and collapse, causing the spine to curve and produce a hunched back. The condition, Pott disease, is now known to result from infection with the tuberculosis organism *Mycobacterium tuberculosis*.

Peyton Rous

(b. Oct. 5, 1879, Baltimore, Md., U.S.—d. Feb. 16, 1970, New York, N.Y.)

American pathologist Peyton Rous was known for his discovery of cancer-inducing viruses. His work earned him a share of the Nobel Prize for Physiology or Medicine in 1966.

Rous was educated at Johns Hopkins University, Baltimore, and at the University of Michigan. He joined the Rockefeller Institute for Medical Research (now Rockefeller University) in New York City in 1909 and remained there throughout his career. In 1911 Rous found that sarcomas in hens could be transmitted to fowl of the same inbred stock not only by grafting tumour cells but also by injecting a submicroscopic agent extractable from them. This discovery gave rise to the virus theory of cancer causation. Although his research was derided at the time, subsequent experiments vindicated his thesis, and he received belated recognition in 1966 when he was awarded (with Charles B. Huggins) the Nobel Prize. Aside from cancer research, Rous did investigations of liver and gallbladder physiology, and he worked on the development of blood-preserving techniques that made the first blood banks possible.

Elizabeth Stern

(b. Sept. 19, 1915, Cobalt, Ont., Can.—d. Aug. 18, 1980, Los Angeles, Calif., U.S.)

Canadian-born American pathologist Elizabeth Stern was noted for her work on the stages of a cell's progression from a normal to a cancerous state.

Stern received a medical degree from the University of Toronto in 1939 and the following year went to the United States, where she became a naturalized citizen in 1943. She received further medical training at the Pennsylvania Medical School and at the Good Samaritan and Cedars of Lebanon hospitals in Los Angeles. She was one of the first specialists in cytopathology, the study of diseased cells. From 1963 she was professor of epidemiology in the School of Public Health at the University of California, Los Angeles.

While at UCLA, Stern became interested in cervical cancer, and she began to focus her research solely on its causes and progression. The discoveries she made during this period led her to publish in 1963 what is believed to be the first case report linking a specific virus (herpes simplex virus) to a specific cancer (cervical cancer). For another phase of her research she studied a group of more than 10,000 Los Angeles county women who were clients of the county's public family planning clinics. In a 1973 article in the journal *Science*, Stern became the first person to report a definite link between the prolonged use of oral contraceptives and cervical cancer. Her research connected the use of contraceptive pills containing steroids with cervical dysplasia, which is often a precursor of cervical cancer. In her most noted work in this field, Stern studied cells cast off from the lining of the cervix and discovered that a normal cell goes through 250 distinct stages of cell progression before reaching an advanced stage of cervical cancer. This prompted the development of diagnostic techniques and screening instruments to detect the cancer in its early stages. Her research helped make cervical cancer, with its slow rate of metastasis, one of the types of cancer that can be successfully treated by prophylactic measures (i.e., excision of abnormal tissue). Stern continued her teaching and research into the late 1970s, despite undergoing chemotherapy for stomach cancer. She died of the disease in 1980.

E. DONNALL THOMAS
(b. March 15, 1920, Mart, Texas, U.S.)

American physician E. Donnall Thomas was famous for his work in transplanting bone marrow from one person to another—an achievement related to the treatment of patients with leukemia and other blood cancers or blood diseases. His work led to his being a corecipient (with Joseph E. Murray) of the 1990 Nobel Prize for Physiology or Medicine.

Thomas studied at the University of Texas (B.A., 1941; M.A., 1943) and the Harvard Medical School (M.D., 1946). He served at a few hospitals and a research centre before becoming a professor of medicine at Columbia University's College of Physicians and Surgeons (1955–63) and the University of Washington School of Medicine (from 1963) in Seattle, where he was also associated with the Fred Hutchinson Cancer Research Center.

In 1956 Thomas performed the first successful bone marrow transplant between two humans: a leukemic patient and his identical twin. The recipient's body accepted the donated marrow and used it to make new, healthy blood cells and immune system cells. Thomas adopted methods to match the tissues of donor and recipient closely enough to minimize the latter's rejection of the former's marrow, and he also developed drugs to suppress the immune system. In 1969 these refinements enabled him to perform the first successful bone marrow transplant in a leukemia patient from a relative who was not an identical twin. Before his work, leukemia had invariably been a fatal disease. By 1990, partially as a result of his research, more than half of all leukemia patients could be expected to survive.

In 1990 Thomas was awarded the U.S. National Medal of Science. Thomas also wrote several books during his career, including *Aplastic Anemia* (1978), *Frontiers on Bone Marrow Transplantation: Fetal Hematopoiesis* (1991), and *Hematopoietic Cell Transplantation* (1999; cowritten with Stephen J. Forman and Karl G. Blume).

HAROLD VARMUS
(b. Dec. 18, 1939, Oceanside, N.Y., U.S.)

American virologist Harold Varmus contributed to work on the origins of cancer. He was a cowinner (with J. Michael Bishop) of the Nobel Prize for Physiology or Medicine in 1989.

Varmus graduated from Amherst (Mass.) College (B.A.) in 1961, from Harvard University (M.A.) in 1962, and from Columbia University, New York City (M.D.), in 1966. He then joined the National Cancer Institute, Bethesda, Md., where he studied bacteria. In 1970 he went to the University of California, San Francisco, as a postdoctoral fellow. There he and Bishop began the research that was to win them the Nobel Prize.

Varmus and Bishop found that, under certain circumstances, normal genes in healthy cells of the body can cause cancer. These genes are called oncogenes. Oncogenes ordinarily control cellular growth and division, but, if they are picked up by infecting viruses or affected by chemical carcinogens, they can be rendered capable of causing cancer. This research, carried out with the aid of colleagues Dominique Stehelin and Peter Vogt in the mid-1970s, superseded a theory that cancer is caused by viral genes, distinct from a cell's normal genetic material, that lie dormant in body cells until activated by carcinogens.

Varmus remained on the faculty of the University of California, where he became a professor of biochemistry and biophysics in 1982. That same year he received an Albert Lasker Basic Medical Research Award for his investigations into the molecular genetics of cancer. He was director of the National Institutes of Health from 1993 to 1999, during which time he significantly increased the budget provided for research. In January 2000 Varmus was appointed president of Memorial Sloan-Kettering Cancer Center in New York City, and he subsequently founded the Public Library of Science (PLoS), a nonprofit organization dedicated to making medical and scientific literature freely available to the public. Varmus was a leading supporter of open-access journals and an advisor for Scientists and Engineers for America, a community of researchers and medical doctors committed to calling attention to science issues on a political level.

In 2001 Varmus was awarded the National Medal of Science for his work on oncogenes and for his work to revitalize scientific research in the United States. Varmus published numerous research papers throughout his career, was a coauthor of *Genes and the Biology of Cancer* (1993; with Robert A. Weinberg), and a coeditor of *Retroviruses* (1997; with John M. Coffin and Stephen H. Hughes).

Rudolf Virchow
(b. Oct. 13, 1821, Schivelbein, Pomerania, Prussia [now Świdwin, Pol.]—d. Sept. 5, 1902, Berlin, Ger.)

German pathologist and statesman Rudolf Virchow was one of the most prominent physicians of the 19th century. He pioneered the modern concept of pathological processes by his application of the cell theory to explain the effects of disease in the organs and tissues of the body. He emphasized that diseases arose, not in organs or tissues in general, but primarily in their individual cells. Moreover, he campaigned vigorously for social reforms and contributed to the development of anthropology as a modern science.

In 1839 Virchow began the study of medicine at the Friedrich Wilhelm Institute of the University of Berlin and was graduated as a doctor of medicine in 1843. As an intern at the Charité Hospital, he studied pathological histology and in 1845 published a paper in which he described one of the two earliest reported cases of leukemia. This paper became a classic.

In 1849 Virchow was appointed to the newly established chair of pathological anatomy at the University of Würzburg—the first chair of that subject in Germany. At Würzburg Virchow published many papers on pathological anatomy. He began there the publication of his six-volume *Handbuch der speziellen Pathologie und Therapie* ("Handbook of Special Pathology and Therapeutics"), most of the first volume of which he wrote himself. At Würzburg he also began to formulate his theories on cellular pathology and started his anthropological work with studies of the skulls of cretins (dwarfed, mentally deficient individuals) and investigations into the development of the base of the skull.

In 1856 a chair of pathological anatomy was established for Virchow at the University of Berlin. During much of this second Berlin period, Virchow actively engaged in politics. In 1859 he was elected to the Berlin City Council, focusing his attention on public health matters, such

as sewage disposal, the design of hospitals, meat inspection, and school hygiene. He supervised the design of two large new Berlin hospitals, the Friedrichshain and the Moabit, opened a nursing school in the Friedrichshain Hospital, and designed the new Berlin sewer system.

In 1861 Virchow was elected to the Prussian Diet. He was a founder of the Fortschrittspartei (Progressive Party) and a determined and untiring opponent of Otto von Bismarck, who in 1865 challenged him to a duel, which he wisely declined. In the wars of 1866 and 1870 Virchow confined his political activities to the erection of military hospitals and the equipping of hospital trains. In the Franco-German War he personally led the first hospital train to the front.

By 1848 Virchow had disproved a prominent view that phlebitis (inflammation of a vein) causes most diseases. He demonstrated that masses in the blood vessels resulted from "thrombosis" (his term) and that portions of a thrombus could become detached to form an "embolus" (also his term). An embolus set free in the circulation might eventually be trapped in a narrower vessel and lead to a serious lesion in the neighbouring parts.

Virchow's concept of cellular pathology was initiated while he was at Würzburg. In the course of his work, he began to realize that one form of the cell theory, which postulated that every cell originated from a preexisting cell rather than from amorphous material,

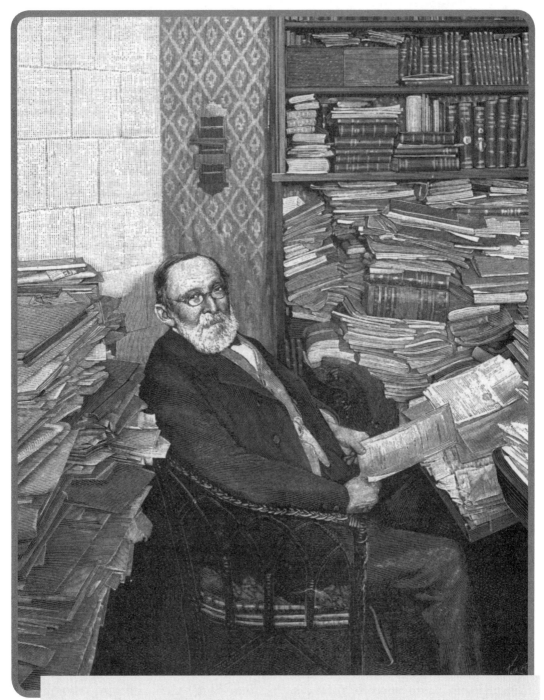

Rudolf Virchow in his office, 1901. © Photos.com/Jupiterimages

could give new insight into pathological processes. In this he was influenced by the work of many others, notably by the views of John Goodsir of Edinburgh on the cell as a centre of nutrition and by the investigations of Robert Remak, a German neuroanatomist and embryologist, who in 1852 was one of the first to point out that cell division accounted for the multiplication of cells to form tissues. By that year Remak had concluded that new cells arose from existing cells in diseased as well as healthy tissue. Remak's writings, however, had little influence on pathologists and medical practitioners. Thus the idea expressed by Virchow's *omnis cellula e cellula* ("every cell is derived from a [preexisting] cell") is not completely original. Even this aphorism is not Virchow's; it was coined by François Vincent Raspail in 1825. But Virchow made cellular pathology into a system of overwhelming importance. His main statement of the theory was given in a series of 20 lectures in 1858. The lectures, published in 1858 as his book *Die Cellularpathologie in ihrer Begründung auf physiologische und pathologische Gewebenlehre* (*Cellular Pathology as Based upon Physiological and Pathological Histology*), at once transformed scientific thought in the whole field of biology.

Virchow shed new light on the process of inflammation, though he erroneously rejected the possibility of migration of the leukocytes (white blood cells). He distinguished between fatty infiltration and fatty degeneration, and he introduced the modern conception of amyloid (starchy) degeneration. He devoted great attention to the pathology of tumours, but the importance of his papers on malignant tumours and of his three-volume work on that subject (*Die krankhaften Geschwülste*, 1863–67) was somewhat marred by his erroneous conception that malignancy results from a conversion (metaplasia) of connective tissue. His work on the role of animal parasites, especially trichina, in causing disease in humans was fundamental and led to his own public interest in meat inspection. In 1874 he introduced a standardized technique for performing autopsies, by the use of which the whole body was examined in detail, often revealing unsuspected lesions.

Virchow's attitude to the new science of bacteriology was complex. He was somewhat resistant to the idea that bacteria had a role in causing disease, and he rightly argued that the presence of a certain microorganism in a patient with a particular disease did not always indicate that that organism was the cause of the disease. He suggested, long before toxins were actually discovered, that some bacteria might produce these substances. Though it is sometimes said that Virchow was antagonistic to Charles Darwin's theory of the origin of species by natural selection, the fact is that he accepted the theory as a hypothesis but maintained throughout his later years that there was insufficient scientific evidence to justify its full acceptance.

BERT VOGELSTEIN
(b. June 2, 1949, Baltimore, Md., U.S.)

American oncologist Bert Vogelstein is known for his groundbreaking work on the genetics of cancer.

Vogelstein was raised in Baltimore and attended a private middle school from which he was often truant, preferring to teach himself by reading at the public library. He received a bachelor's degree in mathematics from the University of Pennsylvania in 1970. Vogelstein then briefly pursued a master's degree in mathematics but instead proceeded to earn a medical degree from the Johns Hopkins University School of Medicine in Baltimore in 1974. He spent the following two years completing his residency in pediatrics at Johns Hopkins Hospital. His experiences working with young cancer patients there influenced his decision to join the National Cancer Institute as a research associate (1976–78). In 1978 he was appointed assistant professor of oncology at Johns Hopkins University.

Although scientists knew that cancer cells were normal cells transformed into unruly mavericks, the reasons for the transformation were unclear until Vogelstein took on the task of elucidating the life history of a tumour cell. In 1982 Vogelstein set out to apply his laboratory expertise to the study of colon cancer. His goal was to identify the genes that, when damaged or defective, give rise to the disease. Analyzing DNA from the cells of colon tumours, he and colleagues found that a particular gene was present in a mutated form in more than one-half of all the tumours they studied. The gene in question, called *K-ras*, belongs to the class known as oncogenes (i.e., cancer-inducing genes). In their normal form, as proto-oncogenes, these genes stimulate cells to replicate when necessary. However, when damaged they may signal the cell to divide ceaselessly. Evidence suggested that a single mutated gene could not trigger the development of cancer. Vogelstein suspected that a defect in another class of growth regulators, called tumour-suppressor genes for their role in preventing uncontrolled cell proliferation, might also be involved. By 1988 his lab had located some of the most frequent chromosomal deletions in colorectal tumours. He became a full professor of oncology at Johns Hopkins in 1989.

Again studying DNA from colon cancer cells, Vogelstein eventually identified three tumour-suppressor genes, *p53* (*TP53*; 1989), *DCC* (1990), and *APC* (1991), mutated forms of which were found in the tumour cells. Further research on *p53* showed that mutations in this gene were involved not only in colon cancer but in a host of other malignancies. In fact, *p53* was implicated in more than 50 percent of all cancerous tumours. Data from Vogelstein's laboratory also provided evidence of still another class of cancer-causing genes, called mismatch repair (MMR) genes, whose normal function is to identify and repair defective

DNA segments. Vogelstein's research made it clear that tumours develop as a result of the sequential accumulation of mutations in proto-oncogenes, tumour-suppressor genes, and mismatch repair genes. On a practical level, his work led to the development of diagnostic tests for colon cancer that promised to greatly reduce deaths from the disease. He later pioneered the use of anaerobic microbes in the treatment of tumours.

In 1992 Vogelstein was elected to the American Academy of Arts and Sciences and the National Academy of Sciences. That year he also received a joint appointment in molecular biology and genetics at Johns Hopkins. In 1995 he became a Howard Hughes Medical Institute investigator and in 1998 was appointed to an additional post in pathology at Johns Hopkins.

In addition to publishing hundreds of articles in professional journals, Vogelstein cowrote *The Genetics of Cancer* (1997) with American oncologist Kenneth Kinzler, one of his former research assistants and later a full professor at Johns Hopkins. Vogelstein was awarded the 1997 William Beaumont Prize for his work on the genetics of cancer.

CHAPTER 7

SURGERY IN THE 20TH CENTURY AND BEYOND

Three seemingly insuperable obstacles beset the surgeon in the years before the mid-19th century: pain, infection, and shock. Once these were overcome, the surgeon believed that he could burst the bonds of centuries and become the master of his craft. There is more, however, to anesthesia than putting the patient to sleep. Infection, despite first antisepsis (destruction of microorganisms present) and later asepsis (avoidance of contamination), is still an ever-present menace, and shock continues to perplex physicians. But in the 20th century, surgery progressed farther, faster, and more dramatically than in all preceding ages.

OBSTACLES IN THE DEVELOPMENT OF SURGERY

The shape of surgery that entered the new century was clearly recognizable as the forerunner of today's, blurred and hazy though the outlines may now seem. The operating theatre still retained an aura of the past, when the surgeon played to his audience and the patient was little more than a stage prop. In most hospitals it was a high room lit by a skylight, with tiers of benches rising above the narrow, wooden operating table. The instruments, kept in glazed or wooden cupboards around the walls, were of forged steel, unplated, and with handles of wood or ivory.

The means to combat infection hovered between antisepsis and asepsis. Instruments and dressings were mostly sterilized by soaking them in dilute carbolic acid (or other antiseptic), and the surgeon often endured a gown freshly wrung out in the same solution. Asepsis gained ground fast, however. It had been born in the Berlin clinic of Ernst von Bergmann where, in 1886, steam sterilization had been introduced. Gradually, this led to the complete aseptic ritual, which has as its basis the bacterial cleanliness (as opposed to social cleanliness) of everything that comes in contact with the wound. Hermann Kümmell, of Hamburg, devised the routine of "scrubbing up." In 1890 William Stewart Halsted, of Johns Hopkins University, had rubber gloves specially made for operating, and in 1896 Johannes von Mikulicz-Radecki, a Pole working at Breslau, Ger., invented the gauze mask.

Many surgeons, brought up in a confused misunderstanding of the antiseptic principle—believing that carbolic would

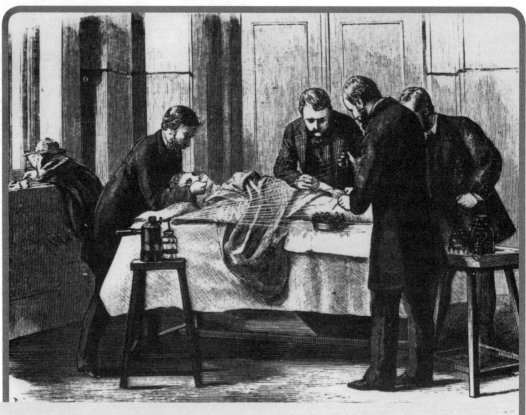

A cloth covered in chloroform is being held over the patient's face, and carbolic spray worked by a steam apparatus is creating an antiseptic atmosphere. Hulton Archive/ Getty Images

cover a multitude of sins, many of which they were ignorant of committing—failed to grasp what asepsis was all about. Thomas Annandale, for example, blew through his catheters to make sure that they were clear, and many an instrument, dropped accidentally, was simply given a quick wipe and returned to use. Tradition died hard, and asepsis had an uphill struggle before it was fully accepted. "I believe firmly that more patients have died from the use of gloves than have ever been saved from infection by their use," wrote W.P. Carr, an American, in 1911. Over the years, however, a sound technique was evolved as the foundation for the growth of modern surgery.

Anesthesia, at the turn of the century, progressed slowly. Few physicians made a career of the subject, and frequently the patient was rendered unconscious by a student, a nurse, or a porter wielding a rag and bottle. Chloroform was overwhelmingly more popular than ether, on account of its ease of administration, despite the fact that it was liable to kill by stopping the heart.

Although by the end of the first decade, nitrous oxide (laughing gas) combined with ether had displaced—but by no means entirely—the use of chloroform, the surgical problems were far from ended. For years to come the abdominal surgeon besought the anesthetist to deepen the level of anesthesia and thus relax the abdominal muscles. The anesthetist responded to the best of his ability, acutely aware that the deeper he went, the closer the patient was to death.

When other anesthetic agents were discovered, the anesthetist came into his own, and many advances in spheres such as brain and heart surgery would have been impossible without his skill.

The third obstacle, shock, is perhaps the most complex and the most difficult to define satisfactorily. The only major cause properly appreciated at the start of the 20th century was loss of blood, and once that had occurred nothing, in those days, could be done. And so, the study of shock—its causes, its effects on human physiology, and its prevention and treatment—became all-important to the progress of surgery.

In the latter part of the 19th century, then, surgeons had been liberated from the age-old bogies of pain, pus, and hospital gangrene. Hitherto, operations had been restricted to amputations, cutting for stone in the bladder, tying off arterial aneurysms (bulging and thinning of artery walls), repairing hernias, and a variety of procedures that could be done without going too deeply beneath the skin. But the anatomical knowledge, a crude skill derived from practice on dead bodies, and above all the enthusiasm, were there waiting. Largely ignoring the mass of problems they uncovered, surgeons launched forth into an exploration of the human body.

They acquired a reputation for showmanship. But much of their surgery, though speedy and spectacular, was rough and ready. There were a few who developed supreme skill and dexterity and could have undertaken a modern operation with but little practice. Indeed, some devised the very operations still in use today. One such was Theodor Billroth, head of the surgical clinic at Vienna, who collected a formidable list of successful "first" operations. He represented the best of his generation—a surgical genius, an accomplished musician, and a kind, gentle man who brought the breath of humanity to his work. Moreover, the men he trained, including von Mikulicz, Vincenz Czerny, and Anton von Eiselsberg, consolidated the brilliant start that he had given to abdominal surgery in Europe.

CHANGES BEFORE WORLD WAR I

The opening decade of the 20th century was a period of transition. Flamboyant exhibitionism was falling from favour as surgeons, through experience, learned the merits of painstaking, conscientious operation—treating the tissues gently and carefully controlling every bleeding point. The individualist was not submerged, however, and for many years the development of the various branches of surgery rested on the shoulders of a few clearly identifiable men. Teamwork on a large scale arrived only after World War II. The surgeon, at first, was undisputed master in his own wards and theatre. But as time went on and he found he could not solve his problems alone, he called for help from specialists in other fields of medicine and, even more significantly, from his colleagues in other scientific disciplines.

The increasing scope of surgery led to specialization. Admittedly, most general surgeons had a special interest, and for a long time there had been an element of specialization in such fields as ophthalmology, orthopedics, obstetrics, and gynecology. But before long it became apparent that, to achieve progress in certain areas, surgeons had to concentrate their attention on that particular subject.

ABDOMINAL SURGERY

By the start of the 20th century, abdominal surgery, which provided the general surgeon with the bulk of his work, had grown beyond infancy, thanks largely to Billroth. In 1881 he had performed the first successful removal of part of the stomach for cancer. His next two cases were failures, and he was stoned in the streets of Vienna. Yet, he persisted and by 1891 had carried out 41 more of these operations with 16 deaths—a remarkable achievement for that era.

Peptic ulcers (gastric and duodenal) appeared on the surgical scene (perhaps as a new disease, but more probably because they had not been diagnosed previously), and in 1881 Ludwig Rydygier cured a young woman of her gastric ulcer by removing it. Bypass operations—gastroenterostomies—soon became more popular, however, and enjoyed a vogue that lasted into the 1930s, even though fresh ulcers at the site of the juncture were not uncommon.

The other end of the alimentary tract was also subjected to surgical intervention. Cancers were removed from the large bowel and rectum with mortality rates that gradually fell from 80 to 60 to 20 to 12 percent as the surgeons developed their skill. In 1908 the British surgeon Ernest Miles carried out the first abdominoperineal resection for cancer of the rectum—the cancer was attacked both from the abdomen and from below through the perineum (the area between the anus and the genitals), either by one surgeon, who actually did two operations, or by two working together. This technique formed the basis for all future developments.

Although much of the new surgery in the abdomen was for cancer, procedures for other conditions were also developed. Appendectomy became the accepted treatment for appendicitis (in appropriate cases) in the United States before the close of the 19th century. But in Great Britain surgeons were reluctant to remove the organ until 1902, when King Edward VII's coronation was dramatically postponed on account of his appendicitis. The publicity attached to his operation caused the disease and its surgical treatment to become fashionable—despite the fact that the royal appendix remained in the King's abdomen. The surgeon, Frederic Treves, had merely drained the abscess.

NEUROSURGERY

Though probably the most demanding of all the surgical specialties, neurosurgery was nevertheless one of the first to emerge. The techniques and principles of general surgery were inadequate for work in such a delicate field. William Macewen, a Scottish general surgeon of outstanding versatility, and Victor Alexander Haden Horsley, the first British neurosurgeon, showed that the surgeon had much to offer in the treatment of disease of the brain and spinal cord. Macewen, in 1893, recorded 19 patients operated on for brain abscess, 18 of whom were cured. At that time most other surgeons had 100 percent mortality rates for the condition. His achievement remained unequaled until the discovery of penicillin.

An American, Harvey Williams Cushing, almost by himself consolidated neurosurgery as a specialty. From 1905 on, he advanced neurosurgery through a series of operations and through his writings. Tumours, epilepsy, trigeminal neuralgia, and pituitary disorders were among the conditions he treated successfully.

RADIOLOGY

In 1895 a development at the University of Würzburg had far-reaching effects on medicine and surgery, opening up an entirely fresh field of the diagnosis and study of disease and leading to a new form of treatment, radiation therapy. This was the discovery of X rays by Wilhelm Conrad Röntgen, a professor of physics. Within months of the discovery there was an extensive literature on the subject: Robert Jones, a British surgeon, had localized a bullet in a boy's wrist before operating; stones in the urinary bladder and gallbladder had been demonstrated; and fractures had been displayed.

Experiments began on introducing substances that are opaque to X rays into the body to reveal organs and formations, both normal and abnormal. Walter Cannon, a Boston physiologist, used X rays in 1898 in his studies of the alimentary tract. Friedrich Voelcker, of Heidelberg, devised retrograde pyelography (introduction of the radiopaque medium into the kidney pelvis by way of the ureter) for the study of the urinary tract in 1905. In Paris in 1921, Jean Sicard X-rayed the spinal canal with the help of an oily iodine substance, and the next year he did the same for the bronchial tree. In 1924 Evarts Graham, of St. Louis, used a radiopaque contrast medium to view the gallbladder. Air was also used to provide contrast. In 1918, at Johns Hopkins, Walter Dandy injected air into the ventricles (liquid-filled cavities) of the brain.

The problems of injecting contrast media into the blood vessels took longer to solve, and it was not until 1927 that António Moniz, of Lisbon, succeeded in obtaining pictures of the arteries of the brain. Eleven years later, George Robb and Israel Steinberg of New York overcame some of the difficulties of cardiac catheterization (introduction of a small tube into the heart by way of veins or arteries) and were able to visualize the chambers of the heart on X-ray film. After much research, a further refinement came in 1962, when Frank Sones and Earl K. Shirey of Cleveland showed how to introduce the contrast medium into the coronary arteries.

SURGERY AND WORLD WAR I

The battlefields of the 20th century stimulated the progress of surgery and taught the surgeon innumerable lessons, which were subsequently applied in civilian practice. Regrettably, though, the principles of military surgery and casualty evacuation, which can be traced back to the Napoleonic wars, had to be learned over again.

World War I broke, quite dramatically, the existing surgical hierarchy and rule of tradition. No longer did the European surgeon have to waste his best years in apprenticeship before seating himself in his master's chair. Suddenly, young surgeons in the armed forces began confronting problems that would have daunted their elders. Furthermore, their training had been in "clean" surgery performed under aseptic conditions. Now they found themselves faced with the need to treat large numbers of grossly contaminated wounds in improvised theatres. They rediscovered debridement (the surgical excision of dead and dying tissue and the removal of foreign matter).

The older surgeons cried "back to Lister," but antiseptics, no matter how strong, were no match for putrefaction and gangrene. One method of antiseptic irrigation—devised by Alexis Carrel and Henry Dakin and called the Carrel–Dakin treatment—was, however, beneficial, but only after the wound had been adequately

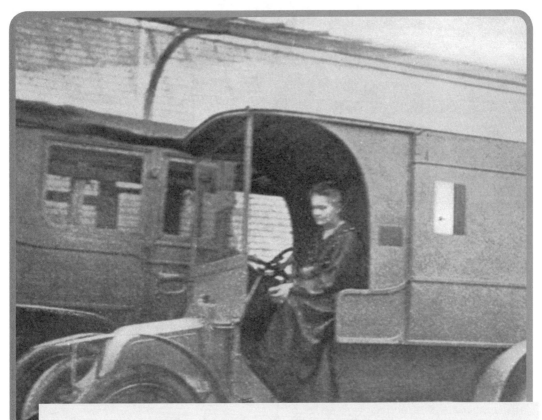

Marie Curie driving a car converted into a mobile radiological unit used to treat wounded soldiers during World War I, 1914. © Photos.Com/Jupiterimages

debrided. The scourges of tetanus and gas gangrene were controlled to a large extent by antitoxin and antiserum injections, yet surgical treatment of the wound remained an essential requirement.

Abdominal casualties fared badly for the first year of the war, because experience in the utterly different circumstances of the South African War had led to a belief that these men were better left alone surgically. Fortunately, the error of continuing with such a policy 15 years later was soon appreciated,

and every effort was made to deliver the wounded men to a suitable surgical unit with all speed. Little progress was made with chest wounds beyond opening up the wound even further to drain pus from the pleural cavity between the chest wall and the lungs.

Perhaps the most worthwhile and enduring benefit to flow from World War I was rehabilitation. For almost the first time, surgeons realized that their work did not end with a healed wound. In 1915 Robert Jones set up special facilities for

DAKIN'S SOLUTION

Dakin's solution (or Carrel-Dakin fluid) is an antiseptic solution containing sodium hypochlorite and developed to treat infected wounds. First used during World War I, Dakin's solution was the product of a long search by an English chemist, Henry Drysdale Dakin, and a French surgeon, Alexis Carrel, for an ideal wound antiseptic.

Stronger germicidal solutions, such as those containing carbolic acid (phenol) or iodine, either damage living cells or lose their potency in the presence of blood serum. Dakin's solution has neither disadvantage. Its solvent action on dead cells hastens the separation of dead from living tissue. Dakin's solution is prepared by passing chlorine into a solution of sodium hydroxide or sodium carbonate. The solution is unstable and cannot be stored more than a few days. The Carrel-Dakin treatment consists of the periodic flooding of an entire wound surface with the solution.

orthopedic patients, and at about the same time Harold Gillies founded British plastic surgery in a hut at Sidcup, Kent. In 1917 Gillies popularized the pedicle type of skin graft (the type of graft in which skin and subcutaneous tissue are left temporarily attached for nourishment to the site from which the graft was taken). Since then plastic surgery has given many techniques and principles to other branches of surgery.

BETWEEN THE WORLD WARS

The years between the two world wars may conveniently be regarded as the time when surgery consolidated its position. A surprising number of surgical firsts and an amazing amount of fundamental research had been achieved even in the late 19th century, but the knowledge and experience could not be converted to practical use because the human body could not survive the onslaught. In the

years between World Wars I and II, it was realized that physiology—in its widest sense, including biochemistry and fluid and electrolyte balance—was of major importance along with anatomy, pathology, and surgical technique.

THE PROBLEM OF SHOCK

The first problem to be tackled was shock, which was, in brief, found to be due to a decrease in the effective volume of the circulation. To combat shock, the volume had to be restored, and the obvious substance was blood itself. In 1901 Karl Landsteiner, then in Austria, discovered the ABO blood groups, and in 1914 sodium citrate was added to freshly drawn blood to prevent clotting. Blood was occasionally transfused during World War I, but three-quarters of a pint was considered a large amount. These transfusions were given by directly linking the vein of a donor with that of the recipient. The continuous drip method, in which blood flows from a flask, was introduced by Hugh Marriott and Alan Kekwick at the Middlesex Hospital, London, in 1935.

As blood transfusions increased in frequency and volume, blood banks were required. Although it took another world war before these were organized on a large scale, the first tentative steps were taken by Sergey Sergeyevich Yudin, of Moscow, who, in 1933, used cadaver blood, and by Bernard Fantus, of Chicago, who, four years later, used living donors as his source of supply. Saline solution, plasma, artificial plasma expanders, and other solutions are now also used in the appropriate circumstances.

Sometimes after operations (especially abdominal operations), the gut becomes paralyzed. It is distended, and quantities of fluid pour into it, dehydrating the body. In 1932 Owen Wangensteen, at the University of Minnesota, advised decompressing the bowel, and in 1934 two other Americans, Thomas Miller and William Abbott, of Philadelphia, invented an apparatus for this purpose, a tube with an inflatable balloon on the end that could be passed into the small intestine. The fluid lost from the tissues was replaced by a continuous intravenous drip of saline solution on the principle described by Rudolph Matas, of New Orleans, in 1924. These techniques dramatically improved abdominal surgery, especially in cases of obstruction, peritonitis (inflammation of the abdominal membranes), and acute emergencies generally, since they made it possible to keep the bowel empty and at rest.

ANESTHESIA AND THORACIC SURGERY

The strides taken in anesthesia from the 1920s onward allowed surgeons much more freedom. Rectal anesthesia had never proved satisfactory, and the first improvement on the combination of nitrous oxide, oxygen, and ether was the introduction of the general anesthetic cyclopropane by Ralph Waters of Madison, Wis., in 1933. Soon afterward, intravenous anesthesia was introduced. John Lundy of the Mayo Clinic brought to a climax a long series of trials by many workers when he used Pentothal (thiopental sodium, a barbiturate) to put a patient peacefully to sleep. Then, in 1942, Harold Griffith and G. Enid Johnson, of Montreal, produced muscular paralysis by the injection of a purified preparation of curare. This was harmless since, by then, the anesthetist was able to control the patient's respiration.

If there was one person who was aided more than any other by the progress in anesthesia, it was the thoracic (chest) surgeon. What had bothered him previously was the collapse of the lung, which occurred whenever the pleural cavity was opened. Since the end of the 19th century, many and ingenious methods had been devised to prevent this from happening. The best known was the negative pressure cabinet of Ernst Ferdinand Sauerbruch, then at Mikulicz' clinic at Breslau. The cabinet was first demonstrated in 1904 but was destined soon to become obsolete.

The solution lay in inhalational anesthesia administered under pressure. Indeed, when Théodore Tuffier, in 1891, successfully removed the apex of a lung for tuberculosis, this was the technique that he used. He even added an inflatable cuff around the tube inserted in the trachea to ensure a gas-tight fit. Tuffier was ahead of his time, however, and other surgeons and research workers wandered into confused and complex byways before Ivan Magill and Edgar Rowbotham, working at Gillies' plastic-surgery unit, found their way back to the simplicity of the endotracheal tube and positive pressure. In 1931 Ralph Waters showed that respiration could be controlled either by squeezing the anesthetic bag by hand or by using a small motor.

These advances allowed thoracic surgery to move into modern times. In the 1920s, operations had been performed mostly for infective conditions and as a last resort. The operations necessarily were unambitious and confined to collapse therapy, including thoracoplasty (removal of ribs), apicolysis (collapse of a lung apex and artificially filling the space), and phrenic crush (which paralyzed the diaphragm on the chosen side); to isolation of the area of lung to be removed by first creating pleural adhesions; and to drainage.

The technical problems of surgery within the chest were daunting until Harold Brunn of San Francisco reported six lobectomies (removals of lung lobes) for bronchiectasis with only one death. (In bronchiectasis one or more bronchi or bronchioles are chronically dilated and inflamed, with copious discharge of mucus mixed with pus.) The secret of Brunn's success was the use of intermittent suction after surgery to keep the cavity free of secretions until the remaining lobes of the lung could expand to fill the space. In 1931 Rudolf Nissen, in Berlin, removed an entire lung from a girl with bronchiectasis. She recovered to prove that the risks were not as bad as had been feared. As far back as 1913 a Welshman, Hugh Davies, removed a lower lobe of the lung for cancer, but a new era began when Evarts Graham removed a whole lung for cancer in 1933. The patient, a doctor, was still alive at the time of Graham's death in 1957.

The thoracic part of the esophagus is particularly difficult to reach, but in 1909 the British surgeon Arthur Evans successfully operated on it for cancer. But results were generally poor until, in 1944, John Garlock, of New York, showed that it is possible to excise the esophagus and to bring the stomach up through the chest and join it to the pharynx. Lengths of colon are also used as grafts to bridge the gap.

WORLD WAR II AND AFTER

Once the principles of military surgery were relearned and applied to modern warfare, instances of death, deformity, and loss of limb were reduced to levels previously unattainable. This was due largely to a thorough reorganization of the surgical services, adapting them to prevailing conditions, so that casualties received the appropriate treatment at the earliest possible moment. Evacuation by air (first used in World War I) helped greatly in this respect. Diagnostic facilities were improved, and progress in anesthesia kept pace with the surgeon's demands. Blood was transfused in adequate—and hitherto unthinkable—quantities, and the blood transfusion service as it is known today came into being.

Surgical specialization and teamwork reached new heights with the creation of units to deal with the special problems of injuries to different parts of the body. But the most revolutionary change was in the approach to wound infections brought about by the use of sulfonamides and (after 1941) of penicillin. The fact that these drugs could never replace meticulous wound surgery was, however, another lesson learned only in the bitter school of experience.

When the war ended, surgeons returned to civilian life feeling that they were at the start of a completely new, exciting era; and indeed they were, for the intense stimulation of the war years had led to developments in many branches of science that could now be applied to surgery. Nevertheless, it must be remembered that these developments merely allowed surgeons to realize the dreams of their fathers and grandfathers. They opened up remarkably few original avenues. The two outstanding phenomena of the 1950s and 1960s—heart surgery and organ transplantation—both originated in a real and practical manner at the turn of the century.

SUPPORT FROM OTHER TECHNOLOGIES

At first, perhaps, the surgeon tried to do too much himself, but before long his failures taught him to share his problems with experts in other fields. This was especially so with respect to difficulties of biomedical engineering and the exploitation of new materials. The relative protection from infection given by antibiotics and chemotherapy allowed the surgeon to become far more adventurous than hitherto in repairing and replacing damaged or worn-out tissues with foreign materials. Much research was still needed to find the best material for a particular purpose and to make sure that it would be acceptable to the body.

Plastics, in their seemingly infinite variety, have come to be used for almost everything from suture material to heart valves; for strengthening the repair of hernias; for replacement of the head of the femur (first done by the French surgeon Jean Judet and his brother Robert-Louis Judet in 1950); for replacement of the lens of the eye after extraction of the natural lens for cataract; for valves to drain fluid from the brain in patients with hydrocephalus; and for many other applications. This is a far cry, indeed, from the unsatisfactory use of celluloid to restore bony defects of the face by the German surgeon Fritz Berndt in the 1890s. Inert metals, such as vitallium, also found a place in surgery, largely in orthopedics for the repair of fractures and the replacement of joints.

The scope of surgery was further expanded by the introduction of the operating microscope. This brought the benefit of magnification particularly to neurosurgery and to ear surgery. In the latter it opened up a whole field of operations on the eardrum and within the middle ear. The principles of these operations were stated in 1951 and 1952 by two German surgeons, Fritz Zöllner and Horst Wullstein. Also in 1952 Samuel Rosen of New York mobilized the footplate of the stapes to restore hearing in otosclerosis—a procedure attempted by the German Jean Kessel in 1876.

Although surgeons aim to preserve as much of the body as disease permits, they are sometimes forced to take radical measures to save life; when, for instance, cancer affects the pelvic organs. Pelvic exenteration (surgical removal of the pelvic organs and nearby structures) in two stages was devised by Allen Whipple of New York City, in 1935, and in one stage by Alexander Brunschwig, of Chicago, in 1937. Then, in 1960, Charles S. Kennedy, of Detroit, after a long discussion with Brunschwig, put into practice an operation that he had been considering for 12 years: hemicorporectomy—surgical removal of the lower part of the body. The patient died on the 11th day. The first successful hemicorporectomy (at the level between the lowest lumbar vertebra and the sacrum) was performed 18 months later by J. Bradley Aust and Karel B. Absolon, of Minnesota. This operation would never have been possible without all the technical, supportive, and rehabilitative resources of modern medicine.

Heart Surgery

The attitude of the medical profession toward heart surgery was for long overshadowed by doubt and disbelief. Wounds of the heart could be sutured (first done successfully by Ludwig Rehn, of Frankfurt am Main, in 1896); the pericardial cavity—the cavity formed by the sac enclosing the heart—could be drained in purulent infections (as had been done by Baron Dominique-Jean Larrey in 1824); and the pericardium could be partially excised for constrictive pericarditis when it was inflamed and constricted the movement of the heart (this operation was performed by Rehn and Sauerbruch in 1913). But little beyond these procedures found acceptance.

Yet, in the first two decades of the 20th century, much experimental work had been carried out, notably by the French surgeons Théodore Tuffier and Alexis Carrel. Tuffier, in 1912, operated successfully on the aortic valve. In 1923 Elliott Cutler of Boston used a tenotome, a tendon-cutting instrument, to relieve a girl's mitral stenosis (a narrowing of the mitral valve between the upper and lower chambers of the left side of the heart) and in 1925, in London, Henry Souttar used a finger to dilate a mitral valve in a manner that was 25 years ahead of its time. Despite these achievements, there was too much experimental failure, and heart disease remained a medical, rather than surgical, matter.

Resistance began to crumble in 1938, when Robert Gross successfully tied off a persistent ductus arteriosus (a fetal blood vessel between the pulmonary artery and the aorta). It was finally swept aside in World War II by the remarkable record of Dwight Harken, who removed 134 missiles from the chest—13 in the heart chambers—without the loss of one patient.

After the war, advances came rapidly, with the initial emphasis on the correction or amelioration of congenital defects. Gordon Murray, of Toronto, made full use of his amazing technical ingenuity to devise and perform many pioneering operations. And Charles Bailey of Philadelphia, adopting a more orthodox approach, was responsible for establishing numerous basic principles in the growing specialty.

Until 1953, however, the techniques all had one great disadvantage: they were done "blind." The surgeon's dream was to stop the heart so that he could see what he was doing and be allowed more time in which to do it. In 1952 this dream began to come true when Floyd Lewis, of Minnesota, reduced the temperature of the body so as to lessen its need for oxygen while he closed a hole between the two upper heart chambers, the atria. The next year John Gibbon, Jr., of Philadelphia, brought to fulfillment the research he had begun in 1937. He used his heart–lung machine to supply oxygen while he closed a hole in the septum between the atria.

Unfortunately, neither method alone was ideal, but intensive research and development led, in the early 1960s, to their being combined as extracorporeal cooling. That is, the blood circulated through a machine outside the body, which cooled it (and, after the operation, warmed it). The cooled blood lowered the temperature of the whole body. With the heart dry and motionless, the surgeon operated on the coronary arteries, inserting plastic patches over holes and sometimes almost remodeling the inside of the heart. But when it came to replacing valves destroyed by disease, surgeons were faced with a difficult choice between human tissue and human-made valves, or even valves from animal sources.

ORGAN TRANSPLANTATION

In 1967 surgery arrived at a climax that made the whole world aware of its medicosurgical responsibilities when the South African surgeon Christiaan Barnard transplanted the first human heart. Reaction, both medical and lay, contained more than an element of hysteria. Yet, in 1964, James Hardy, of the University of Mississippi, had transplanted a chimpanzee's heart into a man, and in that year two prominent research workers, Richard Lower and Norman E. Shumway, had written: "Perhaps the cardiac surgeon should pause while society becomes accustomed to resurrection of the mythological chimera." Research had been remorselessly leading up to just such an operation ever since Charles Guthrie and Alexis Carrel, at the University of Chicago, perfected the suturing of blood vessels in 1905 and then carried out experiments in the transplantation of many organs, including the heart.

Developments in immunosuppression (the use of drugs to prevent organ rejection) advanced the field of transplantation enormously. Kidney transplantation became a routine procedure supplemented by dialysis with an artificial kidney (invented by Willem Kolff in wartime Holland) before and after the operation. Mortality was reduced to about 10 percent per year because of this approach. Rejection of the transplanted heart by the patient's immune system was overcome to some degree in the 1980s with the introduction of the immunosuppressant cyclosporine. Records show that many patients have lived for five or more years after the transplant operation.

The complexity of the liver and the unavailability of supplemental therapies such as the artificial kidney contributed to the slow progress in liver transplantation (first performed in 1963 by Thomas Starzl). An increasing number of patients, especially children, have undergone successful transplantation. However, a substantial number may require retransplantation due to the failure of the first graft.

Lung transplants (first performed by Hardy in 1963) are difficult procedures, and only marginal progress was made in preventing rejection. A combined heart-lung transplant was met with increasing success. Two-thirds of those receiving transplants survived, although complications such as infection are still common.

Transplantation of all or part of the pancreas was not completely successful, and further refinements of the procedures (first performed in 1966 by Richard Lillehei) were needed.

CONTEMPORARY SURGERY

Contemporary surgical therapy is greatly helped by monitoring devices that are used during surgery and during the postoperative period. Blood pressure and pulse rate are monitored during an operation because a fall in the former and a rise in the latter give evidence of a critical loss of blood. Other items monitored are the heart contractions as indicated by electrocardiograms; tracings of brain waves recorded by electroencephalograms, which reflect changes in brain function; the oxygen level in arteries and veins; carbon dioxide partial pressure in the circulating blood; and respiratory volume and exchange. Intensive monitoring of the patient usually continues into the critical postoperative stage.

Asepsis, the freedom from contamination by pathogenic organisms, requires that all instruments and dry goods coming in contact with the surgical field be sterilized. This is accomplished by placing the materials in an autoclave, which subjects its contents to a period of steam under pressure. Chemical sterilization of some instruments is also used. The patient's skin is sterilized by chemicals, and members of the surgical team scrub their hands and forearms with antiseptic or disinfectant soaps. Sterilized gowns, caps, and masks that filter the team's exhaled air and sterilized gloves of disposable plastic complete the picture. Thereafter, attention to avoiding contact with nonsterilized objects is the basis of maintaining asepsis.

During an operation, hemostasis (the arresting of bleeding) is achieved by use of the hemostat, a clamp with ratchets that grasps blood vessels or tissue. After application of hemostats, suture materials are tied around the bleeding vessels. Absorbent sterile napkins called sponges, made of a variety of natural and synthetic materials, are used for drying the field. Bleeding may also be controlled by electrocautery, the use of an instrument heated with an electric current to cauterize, or burn, vessel tissue. The most commonly used instruments in surgery are still the scalpel (knife), hemostatic forceps, flexible tissue-holding forceps, wound retractors for exposure, crushing and noncrushing clamps for intestinal and vascular surgery, and the curved needle for working in depth.

The most common method of closing wounds is by sutures. There are two basic types of suture materials; absorbable ones such as catgut (which comes from sheep intestine) or synthetic substitutes; and nonabsorbable materials, such as nylon sutures, steel staples, or adhesive tissue tape. Catgut is still used extensively to tie off small blood vessels that are bleeding, and since the body absorbs it over time, no foreign materials are left in the wound to become a focus for disease organisms. Nylon stitches and steel staples are removed when sufficient healing has taken place.

There are three general techniques of wound treatment; primary intention, in which all tissues, including the skin, are closed with suture material after completion of the operation; secondary intention, in which the wound is left open and closes naturally; and third intention, in which the wound is left open for a number of days and then closed if it is found to be clean. The third technique is used in badly contaminated wounds to allow drainage and thus avoid the entrapment of microorganisms. Military surgeons use this technique on wounds contaminated by shell fragments, pieces of clothing, and dirt.

The 20th century witnessed several new surgical technologies to supplement the techniques of manual incision. Lasers are now widely used to destroy tumours and other pigmented lesions, some of which are inaccessible by conventional surgery. They are also used to surgically weld detached retinas back in place and to coagulate blood vessels to stop them from bleeding. Stereotaxic surgery uses a three-dimensional system of coordinates obtained by X-ray photography to accurately focus high-intensity radiation, cold, heat, or chemicals on tumours located deep in the brain that could not otherwise be reached. Cryosurgery uses extreme cold to destroy warts and precancerous and cancerous skin lesions and to remove cataracts. In the late 20th century, some traditional techniques of open surgery were being replaced by the use of a thin, flexible fibre-optic tube equipped with a light and a video connection. The tube, or endoscope, is inserted into various bodily passages and provides views of the interior of hollow organs or vessels. Accessories added to the endoscope allow small surgical procedures to be executed inside the body without making a major incision.

Preoperative and postoperative care both have the same object: to restore patients to as near their normal physiologic state as possible. Blood transfusions, intravenous administration of fluids, and the use of measures to prevent common complications such as lung infection and blood clotting in the legs are the principal features of postoperative care.

There are four major categories of surgery: (1) wound treatment, (2) extirpative surgery, (3) reconstructive surgery, and (4) transplantation surgery. The technical aspects of wound surgery, already partly discussed, centre on procuring good healing and the avoidance of infection. Extirpative surgery involves the removal of diseased tissue or organs. Cancer surgery usually falls into this category, with mastectomy (removal of the breast), cholecystectomy (removal of the gallbladder), and hysterectomy (removal of the uterus) among the most frequent procedures. Reconstructive surgery deals with the replacement of lost tissues, whether from fractures, burns, or degenerative-disease processes, and is especially prominent in the practice of plastic surgery and orthopedic surgery. Grafts from the patient or

from others are frequently used to replace lost tissues. Reconstructive surgery also uses artificial devices (prostheses) to replace damaged or diseased organs or tissues. Common examples are the use of metal in reconstructing hip joints and the use of plastic valves to replace heart valves. Transplantation surgery involves the use of organs transplanted from other bodies to replace diseased organs in patients. Kidneys are the most commonly transplanted organs.

The major medical specialties involving surgery are general surgery, plastic surgery, orthopedic surgery, obstetrics and gynecology, neurosurgery, thoracic surgery, colon and rectal surgery, otolaryngology, ophthalmology, and urology. General surgery is the parent specialty and now centres on operations involving the stomach, intestines, breast, blood vessels in the extremities, endocrine glands, tumours of soft tissues, and amputations. Plastic surgery is concerned with the bodily surface and with reconstructive work of the face and exposed parts. Orthopedic surgery deals with the bones, tendons, ligaments, and muscles. Fractures of the extremities and congenital skeletal defects are common targets of treatment. Obstetricians perform cesarean sections, while gynecologists operate to remove tumours from the uterus and ovaries. Neurosurgeons operate to remove brain tumours, treat injuries to the brain resulting from skull fractures, and treat ruptured intravertebral disks that affect the spinal cord.

Thoracic surgeons treat disorders of the lungs; the subspecialty of cardiovascular surgery is concerned with the heart and its major blood vessels and has become a major field of surgical endeavour. Colon and rectal surgery deals with disorders of the large intestine. Otolaryngologic surgery is performed in the area of the ear, nose, and throat (e.g., tonsillectomy), while ophthalmologic surgery deals with disorders of the eyes. Urologic surgery treats diseases of the urinary tract and, in males, of the genital apparatus.

NOTABLE FIGURES IN SURGERY FROM THE 19TH CENTURY TO TODAY

There were many surgeons who performed medical "firsts" in the 19th and 20th centuries. While some of these individuals were known for their innovative approaches to organ transplantation, others introduced new techniques or refined existing ones for operations such as abdominal surgery or neurosurgery. Among the best-known surgeons of these periods are South African surgeon Christiaan Barnard and Viennese surgeon Theodor Billroth.

CHRISTIAAN BARNARD
(b. Nov. 8, 1922, Beaufort West, South Africa—d. Sept. 2, 2001, Paphos, Cyprus)

South African surgeon Christiaan Barnard performed the first human heart transplant operation.

As a resident surgeon at Groote Schuur Hospital, Cape Town (1953–56), Barnard was the first to show that intestinal atresia, a congenital gap in the small intestine, is caused by an insufficient blood supply to the fetus during pregnancy. This discovery led to the development of a surgical procedure to correct the formerly fatal defect. After completing doctoral studies at the University of Minnesota (1956–58), he returned to the hospital as senior cardiothoracic surgeon, introduced open-heart surgery to South Africa, developed a new design for artificial heart valves, and began extensive experimentation on heart transplantation in dogs.

On Dec. 3, 1967, Barnard led a team of 20 surgeons in replacing the heart of Louis Washkansky, an incurably ill South African grocer, with a heart taken from a fatally injured accident victim. Although the transplant itself was successful, Washkansky died 18 days later from double pneumonia, contracted after destruction of his body's immunity mechanism by drugs administered to suppress rejection of the new heart as a foreign protein.

Barnard's later transplant operations were increasingly successful; by the late 1970s a number of his patients had survived for several years. Barnard served as the head of the cardiac unit at Groote Schuur Hospital until 1983, at which time he retired from active surgical practice. He wrote several novels and two autobiographies, *Christiaan Barnard: One Life* (1969) and *The Second Life* (1993).

THEODOR BILLROTH

(b. April 26, 1829, Bergen auf Rügen,
Prussia [Germany]—d. Feb. 6, 1894,
Abbazia, Austria-Hungary [now Opatija,
Croatia])

Viennese surgeon Theodor Billroth is generally considered to be the founder of modern abdominal surgery.

Billroth's family was of Swedish origin. He studied at the universities of Greifswald, Göttingen, and Berlin, Germany, and received his degree from the last in 1852. From 1853 to 1860 he was assistant in B.R.K. Langenbeck's surgical clinic in Berlin, and in 1860 he received the double appointment of regular professor of surgery and director of the surgical clinic at the University of Zürich, Switzerland.

While at Zürich (1860–67), Billroth published his classic *Allgemeine chirurgische Pathologie und Therapie* (1863; *General Surgical Pathology and Therapeutics*). After he joined the faculty at the University of Vienna (1867–94), founding a surgical clinic in the city, he began making major contributions to the practice. He was a pioneer in the study of the bacterial causes of wound fever, as evidenced by *Untersuchungen über die Vegetationsformen von Coccobacteria septica* (1874; "Investigations of the Vegetal Forms of *Coccobacteria septica*"), and was quick to use antiseptic techniques in his surgical practice. With the threat of fatal surgical infections lessened through his work and others', Billroth proceeded to alter or remove organs that had previously been considered inaccessible.

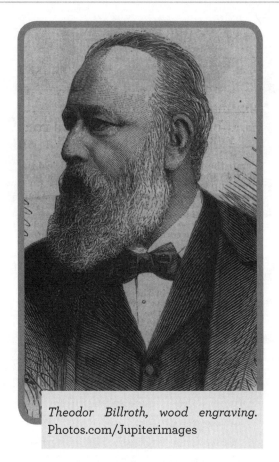

Theodor Billroth, wood engraving. Photos.com/Jupiterimages

In 1872 he was first to remove a section of the esophagus, joining the remaining parts together; a year later he performed the first complete excision of a larynx.

By 1881 he had made intestinal surgery seem almost commonplace and was ready to attempt what appeared in his time as the most formidable abdominal operation conceivable: excision of a cancerous pylorus (the lower end of the stomach). His successful execution of the operation helped to initiate the modern era of surgery. He was also a man of strong artistic bent and was a lifelong friend of the composer Johannes Brahms.

DENTON A. COOLEY
(b. Aug. 22, 1920, Houston, Texas, U.S.)

American surgeon and educator Denton A. Cooley was chiefly noted for heart transplant operations. He was also the first to implant an artificial heart in a human. In April 1969 Cooley observed that the heart of a 47-year-old patient would not function adequately after he removed a section of diseased heart muscle. He implanted a mechanical heart made of silicone, which served as a substitute organ for 65 hours until a heart from a human donor was inserted to replace it. Nevertheless, the patient died 38 hours after the second operation because of pneumonia and kidney failure.

Cooley received an M.D. degree from Johns Hopkins University, Baltimore (1944), and joined the medical faculty of Baylor University College of Medicine, Houston, in 1954. In 1969 he left Baylor to found the Texas Heart Institute, of which he became president and surgeon in chief, and from 1975 he served also as professor of clinical surgery at the University of Texas Medical School in Houston. In 1998 Cooley received the National Medal of Technology, the highest honour for technological innovation.

HARVEY WILLIAMS CUSHING
(b. April 8, 1869, Cleveland, Ohio, U.S.—d. Oct. 7, 1939, New Haven, Conn.)

American surgeon Harvey Williams Cushing was the leading neurosurgeon of the early 20th century.

Cushing graduated from Harvard Medical School in 1895 and then studied for four years at Johns Hopkins Hospital, Baltimore, under William Stewart Halsted. He was a surgeon at Johns Hopkins from 1902 to 1912 and thenceforth was surgeon-in-chief at the Peter Bent Brigham Hospital in Boston and professor of surgery at the Harvard Medical School. In 1933 he joined the faculty of Yale University.

Cushing developed many of the operating procedures and techniques that are still basic to the surgery of the brain, and his work greatly reduced the high mortality rates that had formerly been associated with brain surgery. He became the leading expert in the diagnosis and treatment of intracranial tumours. His research on the pituitary body (1912) gained him an international reputation, and he was the first to ascribe to pituitary malfunction a type of obesity of the face and trunk now known as Cushing disease, or Cushing syndrome. He wrote numerous scientific works and received the Pulitzer Prize in 1926 for his *Life of Sir William Osler* (1925).

MICHAEL DEBAKEY
(b. Sept. 7, 1908, Lake Charles, La., U.S.—d. July 11, 2008, Houston, Texas)

Michael DeBakey was an American cardiovascular surgeon, educator, international medical statesman, and pioneer in surgical procedures for the treatment of defects and diseases of the cardiovascular system.

In 1932 DeBakey devised the "roller pump," an essential component of the heart-lung machine that permitted open-heart surgery. He also developed an efficient method of correcting aortic aneurysms by grafting frozen blood vessels to replace diseased vessels. By 1953 DeBakey had developed a technique of using plastic tubing (Dacron) instead of arterial homographs to replace diseased vessels. In 1953 he performed the first successful carotid endarterectomy for stroke, in 1964 the first successful coronary artery bypass, and in 1966 the first successful implantation of a ventricular assist device.

DeBakey received his B.S. (1930), M.D. (1932), and M.S. (1935) degrees from Tulane University School of Medicine in New Orleans. After volunteering for military service during World War II, his work with the U.S. Surgeon General's office led to the development of mobile army surgical hospitals (MASH units) and the Department of Veterans Affairs (VA) hospital research system. In 1948 he became professor of surgery and chairman of the department of surgery at Baylor College of Medicine in Houston, where he later served as president (1969–79) and then as chancellor (1979–96).

DeBakey received numerous national and international awards, including the American Medical Association Distinguished Service Award (1959), the Albert Lasker Award for Clinical Research (1963; co-recipient), the Eleanor Roosevelt Humanities Award (1969), the Presidential Medal of Freedom with Distinction (1969), the U.S.S.R. Academy of Sciences 50th Anniversary Jubilee Medal (1973), and the Presidential National Medal of Science (1987). He received more than 50 honorary degrees from universities throughout the world. In 1992 he was introduced into the Academy of Athens, a society of scholars generally restricted to Greeks who have made significant contributions to the arts, sciences, or literature. He edited the *Yearbook of Surgery* (1958–70), was the founding editor of the *Journal of Vascular Surgery*, and served on many medical editorial boards. Among his more than 1,600 professional and lay publications is the *The New Living Heart* (1997). DeBakey later received the Denton A. Cooley Cardiovascular Surgical Society's lifetime achievement award (2007) and was bestowed with the highest and most distinguished civilian award given by the U.S. Congress, the Congressional Gold Medal of Honor (2008).

CLARENCE DENNIS
(b. June 16, 1909, St. Paul, Minn., U.S.—d. July 11, 2005, St. Paul)

American surgeon Clarence Dennis performed on April 5, 1951, the world's first open-heart surgery carried out with the use of a heart-lung machine that he had developed at the University of Minnesota. Though the patient died, his pioneering work revolutionized the field of cardiovascular surgery. Dennis joined the staff of the State University of New York Downstate Medical Center in Brooklyn in 1951 and remained there for 20 years. He served (1972–74) as director of technological applications at the National Heart and Lung Institute in Bethesda, Md. Dennis also developed a number of surgical instruments.

CHARLES RICHARD DREW
(b. June 3, 1904, Washington, D.C., U.S.—d. April 1, 1950, near Burlington, N.C.)

African American physician and surgeon Charles Richard Drew was an authority on the preservation of human blood for transfusion.

Drew was educated at Amherst College (graduated 1926), McGill University, Montreal (1933), and Columbia University (1940). While earning his doctorate at Columbia in the late 1930s, he conducted research into the properties and preservation of blood plasma. He soon developed efficient ways to process and store large quantities of blood plasma in "blood banks." As the leading authority in the field, he organized and directed the blood-plasma programs of the United States and Great Britain in the early years of World War II, while also agitating the authorities to stop excluding the blood of African Americans from plasma-supply networks.

Drew resigned his official posts in 1942 after the armed forces ruled that the blood of African Americans would be accepted but would have to be stored separately from that of whites. He then became a surgeon and professor of medicine at Freedmen's Hospital, Washington, D.C., and Howard University (1942–50). He was fatally injured in an automobile accident in 1950.

WILLIAM STEWART HALSTED
(b. Sept. 23, 1852, New York, N.Y., U.S.—d. Sept. 7, 1922, Baltimore, Md.)

American pioneer of scientific surgery William Stewart Halsted established at Johns Hopkins University, Baltimore, the first surgical school in the United States.

After graduating in 1877 from the College of Physicians and Surgeons, New York City, Halsted studied for two years in Europe, mainly in Vienna, under the noted German surgeon Theodor Billroth. Returning to New York, Halsted quickly built a successful practice that demanded his services at six hospitals. In 1881, he discovered that blood, once aerated, could be reinfused into a patient's body.

By self-experimentation he developed (1885) conduction, or block, anesthesia (the production of insensibility of a part by interrupting the conduction of a sensory nerve leading to that region of the body), brought about by injecting cocaine into nerve trunks. He fell into a drug addiction that required two years to cure. Halsted continued his research at Johns Hopkins, where he developed original operations for hernia, breast cancer, goitre, aneurysms, and intestinal and gallbladder diseases.

An early champion of aseptic procedures, Halsted introduced (1890) the use of thin rubber gloves that do not impede the delicate touch demanded by surgery. By ensuring completely sterile conditions in the operating room, Halsted's gloves allowed surgical access to all parts of the body. His emphasis on the maintenance of complete homeostasis, or balanced body metabolism, during surgical operations, gentleness in handling living tissue, accurate realignment of severed tissues, and his creation of hospital residencies in training surgeons did much to advance surgery in the United States.

SIR VICTOR HORSLEY
(b. April 14, 1857, London, Eng.—d. July 16, 1916, Amārah, Iraq)

British physiologist and neurosurgeon Sir Victor Horsley was the first to remove a spinal tumour (1887). He also made valuable studies of thyroid activity, rabies prevention, and the functions of localized areas of the brain.

By removing the thyroid glands of monkeys, he was able to establish (1883) the gland's role in determining the body's rate of growth, development, and metabolism and to implicate thyroid malfunction as the cause of myxedema (a condition characterized by dry, waxy swelling) and cretinism. As secretary to a government commission (1886) appointed to study the effectiveness of Louis Pasteur's rabies vaccine, Horsley corroborated Pasteur's results and led the campaign to eradicate the disease in England. He developed operative techniques that made brain surgery a practical reality and, by 1890, was able to report 44 successful operations. He was knighted in 1902. He died of heatstroke while serving as field surgeon for the British Army in Mesopotamia during World War I.

KARL LANDSTEINER
(b. June 14, 1868, Vienna, Austrian Empire [Austria]—d. June 26, 1943, New York, N.Y., U.S.)

Austrian American immunologist and pathologist Karl Landsteiner received the 1930 Nobel Prize for Physiology or Medicine for his discovery of the major blood groups and the development of the ABO system of blood typing that has made blood transfusion a routine medical practice.

After receiving his M.D. in 1891 from the University of Vienna, Landsteiner studied organic chemistry with many notable scientists in Europe, including the German chemist Emil Fischer. In 1897 he returned to the University of Vienna, where he pursued his interest in the emerging field of immunology and in 1901 published his discovery of the human ABO blood group system.

At that time, although it was known that the mixing of blood from two individuals could result in clumping, or agglutination, of red blood cells, the underlying mechanism of this phenomenon was not understood. Landsteiner discovered the cause of agglutination to be an immunological reaction that occurs when antibodies are produced by the host against donated blood cells. This immune response is elicited because blood from different individuals may vary with respect to certain antigens located on the surface of red blood cells. Landsteiner identified three such antigens, which he labeled A, B, and C (later changed to O). A fourth blood type, later named AB, was identified the following year. He found that if a person with one blood type—A, for example—receives blood from an individual of a different blood type, such as B, the host's immune system will not recognize the B antigens on the donor blood cells and thus will consider them to be foreign and dangerous, as it would regard an infectious microorganism. To defend the body from this perceived threat, the host's immune system will produce antibodies against the B antigens, and agglutination will occur as the antibodies bind to the B antigens. Landsteiner's work made it possible to determine blood type and thus paved the way for blood transfusions to be carried out safely. Landsteiner also discovered other blood factors during his career: the M, N, and P factors, which

he identified in 1927 with Philip Levine, and the Rhesus (Rh) system, in 1940 with Alexander Wiener.

In addition to his study of human blood groups, Landsteiner made a number of other important contributions to science. He and the Romanian bacteriologist Constantin Levaditi discovered that a microorganism is responsible for poliomyelitis and laid the groundwork for the development of the polio vaccine. Landsteiner also helped identify the microorganisms responsible for syphilis. However, he considered his greatest work to be his investigations into antigen-antibody interactions, which he carried out primarily at Rockefeller Institute (now called Rockefeller University) in New York City (1922-43). In this research Landsteiner used small organic molecules called haptens—which stimulate antibody production only when combined with a larger molecule, such as protein—to demonstrate how small variations in a molecule's structure can cause great changes in antibody production. Landsteiner summarized his work in *The Specificity of Serological Reactions* (1936), a classic text that helped establish the field of immunochemistry.

Norman E. Shumway
(b. Feb. 9, 1923, Kalamazoo, Mich., U.S.—d. Feb. 10, 2006, Palo Alto, Calif.)

American surgeon and pioneer in cardiac transplantation Norman E. Shumway on Jan. 6, 1968, at the Stanford Medical Center in Stanford, California, performed the first successful human heart transplant in the United States.

Shumway obtained an M.D. degree from Vanderbilt University (1949) and a Ph.D. degree in surgery from the University of Minnesota (1956), where he studied under Owen Harding Wangensteen and Clarence Walton Lillehei, both distinguished innovators in surgery. In 1958 Shumway joined the faculty of the Stanford University School of Medicine.

As a member of Stanford's cardiovascular research surgery program, Shumway began conducting heart transplants on dogs. About one month after South African surgeon Christiaan Barnard performed the world's first human heart transplant, Shumway performed the operation on a 54-year-old man whose heart had been damaged by a virus infection. The surgery was a success, although the patient died 14 days later. The low long-term survival rates—most patients died soon after surgery because of organ rejection or infection—led many doctors to abandon the procedure by the early 1970s. Shumway, however, continued to improve the operation and advanced a drug that prevented organ rejection. Largely through his efforts, heart transplantation became a viable operation in the 1980s.

In 1981 Shumway was part of a team that performed the first successful heart-lung transplant. His other major achievements included such open-heart procedures as the transplantation of valves. In 1974 Shumway helped found the department of cardiothoracic surgery at Stanford, serving as its first chairman until 1993. He retired from surgery in 1993.

DANIEL HALE WILLIAMS
(b. Jan. 18, 1858, Hollidaysburg, Pa., U.S.—d. Aug. 4, 1931, Idlewild, Mich.)

Daniel Hale Williams, an American physician and the founder of Provident Hospital in Chicago, is credited with the first successful heart surgery.

Williams graduated from Chicago Medical College in 1883. He served as surgeon for the South Side Dispensary (1884–92) and physician for the Protestant Orphan Asylum (1884–93). In response to the lack of opportunity for blacks in the medical professions, he founded (1891) the nation's first interracial hospital, Provident, to provide training for black interns and the first school for black nurses in the United States. He was a surgeon at Provident (1892–93, 1898–1912) and surgeon in chief of Freedmen's Hospital, Washington, D.C. (1894–98), where he established another school for black nurses.

It was at Provident Hospital that Williams performed daring heart surgery on July 10, 1893. Although contemporary medical opinion disapproved of surgical treatment of heart wounds, Williams opened the patient's thoracic cavity without aid of blood transfusions or modern anesthetics and antibiotics. During the surgery he examined the heart, sutured a wound of the pericardium (the sac surrounding the heart), and closed the chest. The patient lived at least 20 years following the surgery. Williams' procedure is cited as the first recorded repair of the pericardium. Some sources, however, cite a similar operation performed by H.C. Dalton of St. Louis in 1891.

Williams later served on the staffs of Cook County Hospital (1903–09) and St. Luke's Hospital (1912–31), both in Chicago. From 1899 he was professor of clinical surgery at Meharry Medical College in Nashville, Tenn., and was a member of the Illinois State Board of Health (1889–91). He published several articles on surgery in medical journals. Williams became the only black charter member of the American College of Surgeons in 1913.

CHAPTER 8

NURSING AND INFLUENTIAL NURSES IN HISTORY

Although nursing became established as a health care profession over a gradual period of time, the activities of Florence Nightingale in the 19th century were fundamental to its progress toward widespread recognition. Through the 20th century, nursing grew significantly and eventually came to fulfill a fundamental role in medicine. Indeed, nursing now is vital in providing physical and emotional care to the sick and disabled and in promoting health in all individuals through activities including research, health education, and patient consultation.

Similar to physicians, nurses can choose training for different specialties (e.g., psychiatry, critical care). Nurse-practitioners, clinical nurse specialists, nurse-anesthetists, and nurse-midwives undertake tasks traditionally performed by physicians. Nursing degrees go as high as the doctorate, and staff positions include administration. In addition to health care settings, nurses practice in schools, the military, industry, and private homes. Community (public health) nurses educate the public on topics such as nutrition and disease prevention.

HISTORICAL OVERVIEW OF NURSING

Although the origins of nursing predate the mid-19th century, the history of professional nursing traditionally begins with Florence Nightingale. In Nightingale's era, the nursing of strangers, either in hospitals or in their homes, was not seen as a respectable career for well-bred ladies, who, if they wished to nurse, were expected to do so only for sick family and intimate friends. In a radical departure from these views, Nightingale believed that well-educated women, using scientific principles and informed education about healthy lifestyles, could dramatically improve the care of sick patients. Moreover, she believed that nursing provided an ideal independent calling full of intellectual and social freedom for women, who at that time had few other career options.

For centuries, most nursing of the sick had taken place at home and had been the responsibility of families, friends, and respected community members with reputations as effective healers. During epidemics, such as cholera, typhus, and smallpox, men took on active nursing roles. For example, Stephen Girard, a wealthy French-born banker, won the hearts of citizens of his adopted city of Philadelphia for his courageous and compassionate nursing of the victims of the 1793 yellow fever epidemic.

As urbanization and industrialization spread, those without families to care for them found themselves in hospitals where the quality of nursing care varied enormously. Some patients received excellent care. Women from religious nursing orders were particularly known for the quality of the nursing care they provided in the hospitals they established. Other hospitals depended on recovering patients or hired men and women for the

nursing care of patients. Sometimes this care was excellent, but other times it was deplorable. The unreliability of hospital-based nursing care became a particular problem by the late 19th century, when changes in medical practices and treatments required competent nurses. The convergence of hospitals' needs, physicians' wishes, and women's desire for meaningful work led to a new health care professional: the trained nurse.

Hospitals established their own training schools for nurses. In exchange for lectures and clinical instructions, students provided the hospital with two or three years of skilled free nursing care. This hospital-based educational model had significant long-term implications. It bound the education of nurses to hospitals rather than colleges, a tie that was not definitively broken until the latter half of the 20th century. The hospital-based training model also reinforced segregation in society and in the health care system. For instance, African American student nurses were barred from almost all American hospitals and training schools. They could seek training only in schools established by African American hospitals. Most of all, the hospital-based training model strengthened the cultural stereotyping of nursing as women's work. Only a few hospitals provided training to maintain men's traditional roles within nursing.

Still, nurses transformed hospitals. In addition to the skilled, compassionate care they gave to patients, they established an orderly, routine, and systemized environment within which patients healed. They administered increasingly complicated treatments and medication regimes. They maintained the aseptic and infection-control protocols that allowed more complex and invasive surgeries to proceed. In addition, they experimented with different models of nursing interventions that humanized increasingly technical and impersonal medical procedures.

Outside hospitals, trained nurses quickly became critical in the fight against infectious diseases. In the early 20th century, the newly discovered "germ theory" of disease (the knowledge that many illnesses were caused by bacteria) caused considerable alarm in countries around the world. Teaching methods of preventing the spread of diseases, such as tuberculosis, pneumonia, and influenza, became the domain of the visiting nurses in the United States and the district nurses in the United Kingdom and Europe. These nurses cared for infected patients in the patients' homes and taught families and communities the measures necessary to prevent spreading the infection. They were particularly committed to working with poor and immigrant communities, which often had little access to other health care services. The work of these nurses contributed to a dramatic decline in the mortality and morbidity rates from infectious diseases for children and adults.

At the same time, independent contractors called private-duty nurses cared for sick individuals in their homes. These nurses performed important clinical work and supported families who had the financial resources to afford care, but the unregulated health care labour market left them vulnerable to competition from both untrained nurses and each year's class of newly graduated trained nurses. Very soon, the supply of private-duty nurses was greater than the demand from families. At the turn of the 20th century, nurses in industrialized countries began to establish professional associations to set standards that differentiated the work of trained nurses from both assistive-nursing personnel and untrained nurses. More important, they successfully sought licensing protection for the practice of registered nursing. Later on, nurses in some countries turned to collective bargaining and labour organizations to assist them in asserting their and their patients' rights to improve conditions and make quality nursing care possible.

By the mid-1930s the increasing technological and clinical demands of patient care, the escalating needs of patients for intensive nursing, and the resulting movement of such care out of homes and into hospitals demanded hospital staffs of trained rather than student nurses. By the mid-1950s hospitals were the largest single employer of registered nurses. This trend continues, although as changes in health care systems have reemphasized care at home, a proportionately greater number of nurses work in outpatient clinics, home care, public health, and other community-based health care organizations.

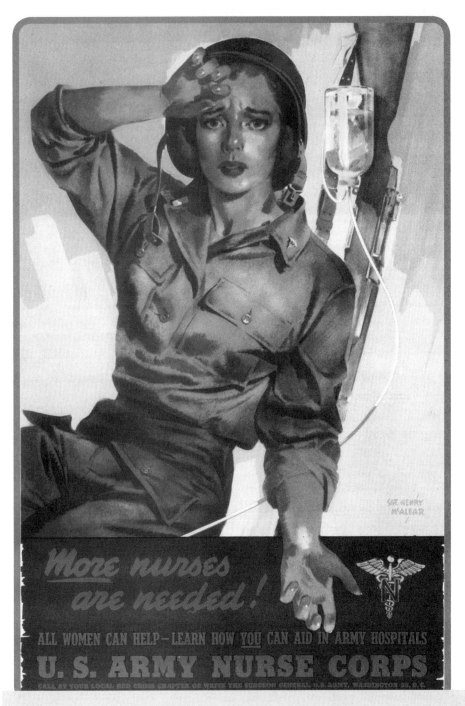

U.S. Army Nurse Corps recruiting poster from World War II. National Library of Medicine, Bethesda, Md.

Other important changes in nursing occurred during the latter half of the 20th century. The profession grew more diverse. For example, in the United States, the National Organization of Coloured Graduate Nurses (NOCGN) capitalized on the acute shortage of nurses during World War II and successfully pushed for the desegregation of both the military nursing corps and the nursing associations. The American Nurses Association (ANA) desegregated in 1949, one of the first national professional associations to do so. As a result, in 1951, feeling its goals fulfilled, the NOCGN dissolved. But by the late 1960s some African American nurses felt that the ANA had neither the time nor the resources to adequately address all their concerns. The National Black Nurses Association (NBNA) formed in 1971 as a parallel organization to the ANA.

Nursing's educational structure also changed. Dependence on hospital-based training schools declined, and those schools were replaced with collegiate programs either in community or technical colleges or in universities. In addition, more systematic and widespread programs of graduate education began to emerge. These programs prepare nurses not only for roles in management and education but also for roles as clinical specialists and nurse practitioners. Nurses no longer had to seek doctoral degrees in fields other than nursing. By the 1970s nurses were establishing their own doctoral programs, emphasizing the nursing knowledge and science and

research needed to address pressing nursing care and care-delivery issues.

During the second half of the 20th century, nurses responded to rising numbers of sick patients with innovative reorganizations of their patterns of care. For example, critical care units in hospitals began when nurses started grouping their most critically ill patients together to provide more effective use of modern technology. In addition, experiments with models of progressive patient care and primary nursing reemphasized the responsibility of one nurse for one patient in spite of the often-overwhelming bureaucratic demands by hospitals on nurses' time.

The nursing profession also has been strengthened by its increasing emphasis on national and international work in developing countries and by its advocacy of healthy and safe environments. The international scope of nursing is supported by the World Health Organization (WHO), which recognizes nursing as the backbone of most health care systems around the world.

FLORENCE NIGHTINGALE
(b. May 12, 1820, Florence [Italy]—d. Aug. 13, 1910, London, Eng.)

Florence Nightingale was a statistician and social reformer and the foundational philosopher of modern nursing. Nightingale was put in charge of nursing British and allied soldiers in Turkey during the Crimean War. She spent many hours in the wards, and her night rounds giving personal care to the wounded established her image as the "Lady with the Lamp." Her efforts to formalize nursing education led her to establish the first scientifically based nursing school—the Nightingale School of Nursing, at St. Thomas' Hospital in London (opened 1860). She also was instrumental in setting up training for midwives and nurses in workhouse infirmaries. She was the first woman awarded the Order of Merit (1907).

Family Ties and Spiritual Awakening

Florence Nightingale was the second of two daughters born, during an extended European honeymoon, to William Edward and Frances Nightingale. (William Edward's original surname was Shore; he changed his name to Nightingale after inheriting his great-uncle's estate in 1815.) Florence was named after the city of her birth. After returning to England in 1821, the Nightingales had a comfortable lifestyle, dividing their time between two homes, Lea Hurst in Derbyshire, located in central England, and Embley Park in warmer Hampshire, located in south-central England. Embley Park, a large and comfortable estate, became the primary family residence, with the Nightingales taking trips to Lea Hurst in the summer and to London during the social season.

Florence was a precocious child intellectually. Her father took particular interest in her education, guiding her through history, philosophy, and literature. She excelled in mathematics and languages and was able to read and write French, German, Italian, Greek, and Latin at an early age. Never satisfied with the traditional female skills of home management, she preferred to read the great philosophers and to engage in serious political and social discourse with her father.

As part of a liberal Unitarian family, Florence found great comfort in her religious beliefs. At the age of 16, she experienced one of several "calls from God." She viewed her particular calling as reducing human suffering. Nursing seemed the suitable route to serve both God and humankind. However, despite having cared for sick relatives and tenants on the family estates, her attempts to seek nurse's training were thwarted by her family as an inappropriate activity for a woman of her stature.

Nursing in Peace and War

Despite family reservations, Nightingale was eventually able to enroll at the Institution of Protestant Deaconesses at Kaiserswerth in Germany for two weeks of training in July 1850 and again for three months in July 1851. There she learned basic nursing skills, the importance of patient observation, and the value of good hospital organization. In 1853 Nightingale sought to break free from her family environment. Through social connections, she became the superintendent of the Institution for Sick Gentlewomen (governesses) in

Distressed Circumstances, in London, where she successfully displayed her skills as an administrator by improving nursing care, working conditions, and efficiency of the hospital. After one year she began to realize that her services would be more valuable in an institution that would allow her to train nurses. She considered becoming the superintendent of nurses at King's College Hospital in London. However, politics, not nursing expertise, was to shape her next move.

In October 1853 the Turkish Ottoman Empire declared war on Russia, following a series of disputes over holy places in Jerusalem and Russian demands to exercise protection over the Orthodox subjects of the Ottoman sultan. The British and the French, allies of Turkey, sought to curb Russian expansion. The majority of the Crimean War was fought on the Crimean Peninsula in Russia. However, the British troop base and hospitals for the care of the sick and wounded soldiers were primarily established in Scutari (Üsküdar), across the Bosporus from Constantinople (Istanbul). The status of the care of the wounded was reported to the London *Times* by the first modern war correspondent, British journalist William Howard Russell. The newspaper reports stated that soldiers were treated by an incompetent and ineffective medical establishment and that the most basic supplies were not available for care. The British public raised an outcry over the treatment of the soldiers and demanded that the situation be drastically improved.

Sidney Herbert, secretary of state at war for the British government, wrote to Nightingale requesting that she lead a group of nurses to Scutari. At the same time, Nightingale wrote to her friend Liz Herbert, Sidney's wife, asking that she be allowed to lead a private expedition. Their letters crossed in the mail, but in the end their mutual requests were granted. Nightingale led an officially sanctioned party of 38 women, departing Oct. 21, 1854, and arriving in Scutari at the Barrack Hospital on November 5. Not welcomed by the medical officers, Nightingale found conditions filthy, supplies inadequate, staff uncooperative, and overcrowding severe. Few nurses had access to the cholera wards, and Nightingale, who wanted to gain the confidence of army surgeons by waiting for official military orders for assistance, kept her party from the wards. Five days after Nightingale's arrival in Scutari, injured soldiers from the Battle of Balaklava and the Battle of Inkerman arrived and overwhelmed the facility. Nightingale said it was the "Kingdom of Hell."

In order to care for the soldiers properly, it was necessary that adequate supplies be obtained. Nightingale bought equipment with funds provided by the London *Times* and enlisted soldiers' wives to assist with the laundry. The wards were cleaned and basic care was provided by the nurses. Most important, Nightingale established standards of care, requiring such basic necessities as bathing, clean clothing and dressings, and adequate food. Attention was given to psychological needs through assistance in writing letters to relatives and through providing educational and recreational activities. Nightingale herself wandered the wards at night, providing support to the patients. This earned her the title of "Lady with the Lamp." She gained the respect of the soldiers and medical establishment alike. Her accomplishments in providing care and reducing the mortality rate to about 2 percent brought her fame in England through the press and the soldiers' letters.

In May 1855 Nightingale began the first of several excursions to the Crimea. However, shortly after arriving, she fell ill with "Crimean fever"—most likely brucellosis, which she probably contracted from drinking contaminated milk. Nightingale experienced a slow recovery, as no active treatment was available. The lingering effects of the disease were to last for 25 years, frequently confining her to bed because of severe, chronic pain.

On March 30, 1856, the Treaty of Paris ended the Crimean War. Nightingale remained in Scutari until the hospitals were ready to close, returning to her home in Derbyshire on Aug. 7, 1856, as a reluctant heroine.

HOMECOMING AND LEGACY

Although primarily remembered for her accomplishments during the Crimean War, Nightingale's greatest achievements centred on attempts to create social reform in health care and nursing.

On her return to England, Nightingale was suffering the effects of both brucellosis and exhaustion. In September 1856 she met with Queen Victoria and Prince Albert to discuss the need for reform of the British military establishment. Nightingale kept meticulous records regarding the running of the Barrack Hospital, causes of illness and death, the efficiency of the nursing and medical staffs, and difficulties in purveyance. A Royal Commission was established, which based its findings on the statistical data and analysis provided by Nightingale. The result was marked reform in the military medical and purveyance systems.

In 1855, as a token of gratitude and respect for Nightingale, the Nightingale Fund was established. Through private donations, £45,000 was raised by 1859 and put at Nightingale's disposal. She used a substantial part of these monies to institute the Nightingale School of Nursing at St. Thomas' Hospital in London, which opened in 1860. The school formalized secular nursing education, making nursing a viable and respectable option for women who desired employment outside of the home. The model was taken worldwide by matrons (women supervisors of public health institutions). Nightingale's statistical models—such as the Coxcomb chart, which she developed to assess mortality—and her basic concepts regarding nursing remain applicable today. For these reasons she is considered the foundational philosopher of modern nursing.

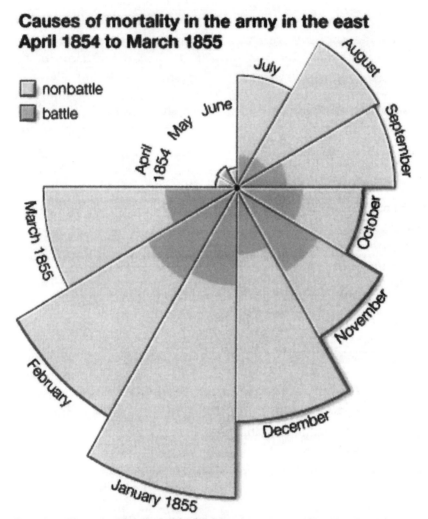

Coxcomb

Causes of mortality in the army in the east April 1854 to March 1855

☐ nonbattle
☐ battle

April 1854 — *May* — *June* — *July* — *August* — *September* — *October* — *November* — *December* — *January 1855* — *February* — *March 1855*

Based on Florence Nightingale's "Notes on Matters Affecting the Health, Efficiency and Hospital Administration of the British Army," 1858.

The English nurse Florence Nightingale was an innovator in displaying statistical data through graphs. In 1858 she devised the type depicted here, which she named the Coxcomb chart. Like pie charts, the Coxcomb indicates frequency by relative area, but it differs in its use of fixed angles and variable radii. Encyclopædia Britannica, Inc.

Nightingale improved the health of households through her most famous publication, *Notes on Nursing: What It Is and What It Is Not*, which provided direction on how to manage the sick. This volume has been in continuous publication worldwide since 1859. Additional reforms were financed through the Nightingale Fund, and a school for the education of midwives was established at King's College Hospital in 1862. Believing that the most important location for the care of the sick was in the home, she established training for district nursing, which was aimed at improving the health of the poor and vulnerable. A second Royal Commission examined the health of India, resulting in major environmental reform, again based on Nightingale's statistical data.

Florence Nightingale was honoured in her lifetime by receiving the title of Lady of Grace of the Order of St. John of Jerusalem and by becoming the first woman to receive the Order of Merit. On her death in 1910, at Nightingale's prior request, her family declined the offer of a state funeral and burial in Westminster Abbey. Instead, she was honoured with a memorial service at St. Paul's Cathedral, London. Her burial is in the family plot in St. Margaret's Church, East Wellow, Hampshire.

MARY ANN BICKERDYKE

(b. July 19, 1817, Knox county, Ohio, U.S.—d. Nov. 8, 1901, Bunker Hill, Kan.)

Mary Ann Bickerdyke (née Mary Ann Ball) was the organizer and chief of nursing, hospital, and welfare services for the western armies under the command of General Ulysses S. Grant during the American Civil War.

Mary Ann Ball grew up in the houses of various relatives. She attended Oberlin College and later studied nursing. In 1847 she married a widower, Robert Bickerdyke, who died in 1859. Thereafter Mary Ann Bickerdyke supported herself in Galesburg, Illinois, by the practice of "botanic" medicine.

Soon after the outbreak of the Civil War, she volunteered to accompany and distribute a collection of supplies taken up for the relief of wounded soldiers at a makeshift army hospital in Cairo, Illinois. On her arrival there she found conditions to be extremely unsanitary, and she set to work immediately at cleaning, cooking, and nursing. She became matron when a general hospital was organized there in November 1861. Following the fall of Fort Donelson in February 1862, she made a number of forays onto the battlefield to search for wounded, and her exploits began to attract general attention. Her alliance with the U.S. Sanitary Commission began about that time.

Bickerdyke soon attached herself to the staff of General Ulysses S. Grant, by whom she was given a pass for free transportation anywhere in his command. She followed Grant's army down the Mississippi River, setting up hospitals as they were needed, and later accompanied the forces of General William Tecumseh Sherman on their march through Georgia to the sea. Through her efforts, provisions were made for frequent medical examinations and for transporting men who could no longer walk. Under Bickerdyke's supervision, about 300 field hospitals were built with the help of U.S. Sanitary Commission agents.

Having scavenged supplies and equipment and established mobile laundries and kitchens, Bickerdyke had generally endeared herself to the wounded and sick, among whom she became known as "Mother" Bickerdyke. To incompetent officers and physicians she was brutal, succeeding in having several dismissed, and she retained her position largely through the influence of Grant, Sherman, and others who recognized the value of her services.

During 1866–67 she worked with the Chicago Home for the Friendless, and in 1867, in connection with a plan to settle veterans on Kansas farmland, she opened a boarding house in Salina with backing from the Kansas Pacific Railroad. The venture failed in 1869, and in 1870 she went to New York City to work for the Protestant Board of City Missions. In 1874 she returned to Kansas, where her sons lived, and made herself conspicuously useful in relieving the victims of locust plague.

In 1876 Bickerdyke removed to San Francisco, where she secured through Senator John A. Logan, another wartime patron, a position at the U.S. Mint. She also devoted considerable time to the Salvation Army and similar organizations. She worked tirelessly on behalf of veterans, making numerous trips to

Washington to press pension claims, and was herself granted a pension of $25 a month by Congress in 1886. She returned to Kansas in 1887 and died there in 1901.

FLORENCE A. BLANCHFIELD
(b. April 1, 1884, Shepherdstown, W.Va., U.S.—d. May 12, 1971, Washington, D.C.)

American nurse and army officer Florence A. Blanchfield succeeded in winning the status of full rank for U.S. Army nurses and became the first woman to hold a regular commission in that military branch.

Blanchfield was educated at business college in Pittsburgh, Pennsylvania, at the University of California, and at Columbia University in New York City. In 1906 she graduated from the South Side Training School for Nurses in Pittsburgh. After additional training at the Johns Hopkins Hospital, Baltimore, Maryland, she entered upon a succession of posts in Pennsylvania and the Canal Zone (1913). In 1917 she enlisted in the Army Nurse Corps, and she served in France until 1919. She subsequently was assigned to army hospitals in Michigan, California, the Philippines, Washington, D.C., Georgia, Missouri, and China. She also served for a time in the office of the surgeon general.

In 1942 she was given a commission as lieutenant colonel to serve as assistant to Colonel Julia Flikke, superintendent of the Army Nurse Corps. Because their ranks were found to be without legal basis, they were paid as major and lieutenant colonel, respectively, and when Blanchfield succeeded Flikke as superintendent in 1943, she made it one of her concerns to secure full rank, as opposed to relative rank (which consisted of the formality but not the pay or benefits of full rank), for army nurses. During World War II Blanchfield supervised the worldwide work of some 60,000 nurses on all fronts. Her case for full rank was won on a temporary basis in 1944, and in April 1947 both the army and the navy revised regulations to permit women to hold full rank. Blanchfield thereupon received from General Dwight D. Eisenhower the first regular army commission to be awarded to a woman. She retired that year and thereafter lived in Arlington, Virginia.

MARY BRECKINRIDGE

(b. Feb. 17, 1881, Memphis, Tenn., U.S.—d. May 16, 1965, Hyden, Ky.)

American nurse-midwife Mary Breckinridge established neonatal and childhood medical care systems in the United States. Her efforts led to dramatic reductions in mortality rates of mothers and infants.

Breckinridge grew up in Washington, D.C., where her father was an Arkansas congressman, and in St. Petersburg, Russia, where he served as U.S. minister to Russia. Educated at private schools in Lausanne, Switzerland, and Stamford, Connecticut, she returned to her family's Arkansas home in 1899. After her 1904 marriage ended in 1906 with her

husband's death, she entered St. Luke's Hospital School of Nursing in New York City, graduating and, in 1910, receiving her R.N. In 1912 she married Richard Ryan Thompson, president of a Eureka Springs, Arkansas, women's school where she taught French and hygiene. Devastated by the deaths of her newborn daughter in 1916 and her four-year-old son in 1918, she decided to honour their memory by devoting her life to improving children's conditions.

Leaving her husband six months before the end of World War I, she worked as a public health nurse in Boston and Washington, D.C., while awaiting a posting with the American Red Cross in France. (She resumed use of her maiden name after her divorce became final in 1920.) Arriving in France after the armistice to work with the American Committee for Devastated France, she initiated a program to provide food and medical assistance for children, nursing mothers, and pregnant women. From her work in France and visits to England she became convinced that the health of rural American children would benefit from the presence of trained midwives.

To prepare to make the goal a reality, she studied public health nursing at Teachers College of Columbia University and midwifery at three British institutions. She also embarked on an educational trip to Scotland, where she observed how a nursing service there effectively provided medical care to a dispersed population. In 1925 she moved to Leslie county, Kentucky, where she founded the Frontier Nursing Service, which she subsidized with her inheritance from her mother. The introduction of nurse-midwives into the region brought its maternal and neonatal death rates well below the national average, and at a reasonable cost. In addition to directing the service, which led to the foundation in 1929 of the American Association of Nurse-Midwives, she also edited its journal and traveled around the country as a fund-raiser. Breckinridge's autobiography, *Wide Neighborhoods: A Story of the Frontier Nursing Service,* was published in 1952.

EDITH CAVELL
(b. Dec. 4, 1865, Swardeston, Norfolk, Eng.—d. Oct. 12, 1915, Brussels, Belg.)

English nurse Edith Cavell became a popular heroine of World War I and was executed for assisting Allied soldiers to escape from German-occupied Belgium.

Cavell entered the nursing profession in 1895 and in 1907 was appointed the first matron of the Berkendael Institute, Brussels, where she greatly improved the standard of nursing. After the German occupation of Belgium, she became involved in an underground group formed to help British, French, and Belgian soldiers reach the Netherlands, a neutral country. The soldiers were sheltered at the Berkendael Institute, which had become a Red Cross hospital, and were provided with money and guides by Philippe Baucq, a Belgian. About 200

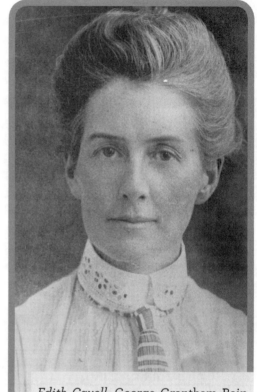

Edith Cavell. George Grantham Bain Collection/Library of Congress, Washington, D.C. (Digital File Number: LC-DIG-ggbain-20235)

men had been aided when, in August 1915, Cavell and several others were arrested.

The group was brought before a court-martial on Oct. 7, 1915. On October 9, Cavell, after making a full confession, was sentenced to death. Three days later she and Baucq were shot, despite the efforts of the U.S. and Spanish ministers to secure a reprieve. Though legally justified, her execution on a charge that did not include espionage was considered outrageous and was widely publicized by the Allies.

SUE SOPHIA DAUSER

(b. Sept. 20, 1888, Anaheim, Calif.,
U.S.—d. March 8, 1972, Anaheim)

American nurse and naval officer Sue Sophia Dauser was responsible for preparing the Navy Nurse Corps for World War II and then overseeing the group, who simultaneously worked for parity of rank and pay for female officers and their male counterparts.

Dauser attended Stanford University from 1907 to 1909 and in 1911 entered the California Hospital School of Nursing, Los Angeles, graduating in 1914. In September 1917 she joined the naval reserve, going on active duty the next month. In July 1918 she entered the regular navy. After duty at Base Hospital No. 3 in Edinburgh during the final months of World War I, she served tours of duty at naval hospitals in Brooklyn, New York, and San Diego, California, and aboard ship. In 1923 she sailed on the *Henderson* on President Warren G. Harding's Alaskan visit and attended him during his last illness. She later served on Guam; in the Philippines; at San Diego, California; in Puget Sound off Washington state; and on Mare Island and at Long Beach, California.

In 1939 Dauser was named superintendent of the Navy Nurse Corps. Her task in that post was twofold: to organize and administer a greatly expanded Nurse Corps in preparation for and then throughout World War II and to secure for navy nurses equitable rank and privileges. In July 1942 Congress provided for relative rank for nurses (title and uniform but not the commission, pay, or other benefits of regular rank), and she became a lieutenant commander. Pay was made equivalent in December 1942. In December 1943 Dauser was promoted to (relative) captain, equivalent to Florence A. Blanchfield's army colonelcy and the highest naval rank yet attained by a woman.

In February 1944 temporary commissions were authorized for army and navy nurses. Captain Dauser retired as superintendent of nurses in November 1945 and was awarded the Distinguished Service Medal soon thereafter. Under Dauser the Navy Nurse Corps had grown from 600 members to 11,500. She lived afterward in retirement in La Mesa, California.

JANE A. DELANO

(b. March 12, 1862, Montour Falls, N.Y.,
U.S.—d. April 15, 1919, Savenay, France)

American nurse and educator Jane A. Delano made possible the enlistment of more than 20,000 U.S. nurses for overseas duty during World War I.

Delano taught school for two years and graduated from the Bellevue Hospital School of Nursing in New York City in 1886. She became superintendent of nurses (1887–88) in Jacksonville, Florida, where she insisted on the use of mosquito netting to prevent the spread of yellow fever at a time when the mosquito was not known to be a carrier of the disease. In Bisbee, Arizona, she established a hospital for the care of miners suffering from scarlet fever.

From 1890 to 1895 Delano was assistant superintendent of nurses and an instructor at the University of Pennsylvania Hospital School of Nursing. Over the next five years she was engaged in a variety of activities and undertook brief courses of study at the University of Buffalo Medical School and the New York School of Civics and Philanthropy. She then directed the girls' department of the New York City House of Refuge on Randall's Island (1900–02) and was superintendent of the nursing schools of Bellevue and its associated hospitals (1902–06). From 1906 to 1908 she was largely out of professional life while she attended her mother in her last illness.

While serving as chairman of the Red Cross national committee on nursing service and as superintendent of the Army Nurse Corps (1909–12), Delano carried out a plan to make the Red Cross Nursing Service the reserve for the corps. As a result, 8,000 nurses were ready for overseas duty when the U.S. entered World War I. During the course of the war, Delano saw to the mobilization of upward of 20,000 nurses, as well as a great number of nurses' aides and other workers, for duty overseas. In 1918 she became director of the wartime organization, the Department of Nursing, which supplied nurses to the army, navy, and Red Cross.

Delano served three terms as president of the American Nurses Association (1900–12) and one as president of the

Board of Directors of the *American Journal of Nursing* (1908–11). She wrote, with Isabel McIsaac, the *American Red Cross Textbook on Elementary Hygiene and Home Care of the Sick* (1913). The influenza epidemic that swept Europe and America in 1918–19 vastly increased the demand for her and the Red Cross's services. Already exhausted by her labours, Delano fell ill and died while on a European inspection tour.

SISTER MARY JOSEPH DEMPSEY

(b. May 14, 1856, Salamanca, N.Y., U.S.—d. March 29, 1939, Rochester, Minn.)

American nurse and hospital administrator Sister Mary Joseph Dempsey (original name Julia Dempsey) was remembered for her exceptional medical and administrative abilities and for her contributions to nursing education.

Julia Dempsey in August 1878 entered the Third Order Regular of St. Francis of the Congregation of Our Lady of Lourdes, taking the name Sister Mary Joseph. She taught school in many places over the next several years before being called to Rochester in 1889 to help staff the new St. Mary's Hospital, built by her order in the wake of a disastrous tornado. The hospital medical staff consisted of the Mayo family—William W. Mayo and his two sons, Charles H. and William J. Mayo. Sister Mary Joseph studied nursing under a local nurse and in 1890 became William J. Mayo's first surgical assistant, a post she held until 1915. In that work she displayed rare skill and judgment. In September 1892 she was also appointed superintendent of St. Mary's Hospital, a task she was to carry on for the rest of her life. During that nearly 40 years, the hospital underwent six major expansions, growing from 45 to 600 beds and in time incorporating the most modern and efficient facilities, particularly for surgery. In 1906 Sister Mary Joseph opened St. Mary's Hospital School for Nurses, which trained both sisters and laywomen. In 1915 she helped organize the Catholic Hospital Association of the United States and Canada and was chosen its first vice president. In addition to her work at St. Mary's, her remarkable administrative and medical skills contributed greatly to the success of the Mayo brothers in establishing their world-famous surgical practice and their Mayo Clinic.

CLARA MAASS

(b. June 28, 1876, East Orange, N.J., U.S.—d. Aug. 24, 1901, Havana, Cuba)

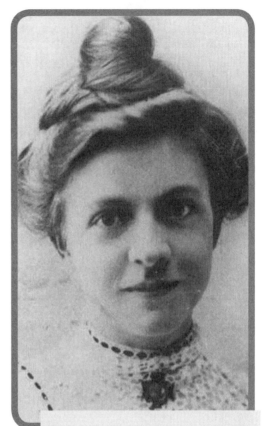

Clara Maass. Office of Medical History

American nurse Clara Maass was the only woman and the only American to die during the yellow fever experiments of 1900–01.

Maass graduated from the Newark (New Jersey) German Hospital School of Nursing in 1895 and shortly afterward was named head nurse of the school. At the outbreak of the Spanish-American War in April 1898, she volunteered to serve as a contract nurse with the U.S. Army Medical Department. During her first term of service she worked at army camps in Florida, Georgia, and Cuba. She volunteered again in 1900 and was sent first to the Philippines and then back to Cuba.

Her long experience in nursing victims of yellow fever drew Maass into the work of the Yellow Fever Commission headed by Major Walter Reed. While at Las Animas Hospital in Havana, Maass volunteered to take part in an experiment conducted by Major William C. Gorgas and John Guitéras on yellow fever immunization. The theory of the experiment was that, given prompt hospital care under controlled conditions, a mild case of yellow fever would ensue and the victim would recover, immune thereafter. Such had been Reed's experience during his classic demonstration that yellow fever is spread exclusively by the mosquito. On Aug. 14, 1901, Maass allowed herself to be bitten by an infected *Stegomyia fasciata* mosquito (later renamed *Aedes aegypti*). Contrary to expectations, however, Maass came down with a severe fever and died 10 days later. In 1952 the Newark German Hospital, which had meanwhile changed its name to Lutheran Memorial, was renamed the Clara Maass Memorial Hospital.

MARY MAHONEY
(b. May 7, 1845, Dorchester, Mass., U.S.—d. Jan. 4, 1926, Boston, Mass.)

American nurse Mary Mahoney was the first African American woman to complete the course of professional study in nursing.

Mahoney apparently worked as a maid at the New England Hospital for Women and Children in Boston before being admitted to its nursing school in 1878. She received her diploma in 1879, becoming the first black woman to complete nurse's training. At the time of her graduation, seriously ill patients were routinely treated at home rather than in a hospital, and Mahoney was employed for many years as a private-duty nurse. One of the first black members of the Nurses Associated Alumnae of the United States and Canada (subsequently renamed the

American Nurses Association, or ANA), she later joined the National Association of Colored Graduate Nurses (NACGN) and addressed its first annual convention in Boston (1909). The association awarded her life membership in 1911 and elected her its national chaplain.

From 1911 to 1912 Mahoney served as supervisor of the Howard Orphan Asylum for Black Children in Kings Park, Long Island, New York. Returning to Boston, she is reputed to have been one of the first women in that city to register to vote after the ratification of the Nineteenth Amendment in 1920. Ten years after her death in 1926, the NACGN honoured her memory by establishing the Mary Mahoney Medal, an award to a member for distinguished service to the profession. After the NACGN merged with the ANA in 1951, the award was continued. It is now conferred bienially on an individual who has made a significant contribution to opening up opportunities in nursing to minorities. Mahoney was named to the Nursing Hall of Fame in 1976 and to the National Women's Hall of Fame in 1993.

LUCY MINNIGERODE
(b. Feb. 8, 1871, near Leesburg, Va., U.S.—d. March 24, 1935, Alexandria, Va.)

American nurse Lucy Minnigerode was noted for her work in organizing nurses for the Red Cross and the U.S. Public Health Service.

Minnigerode was educated in private schools. She studied at the Training

School for Nurses of Bellevue Hospital in New York City (1899–1905) and became a registered nurse in 1905. She was in private practice until 1910, when she became superintendent of nurses at the Episcopal Eye, Ear and Throat Hospital in Washington, D.C. Later she held a similar post at the Savannah (Georgia) Hospital.

In 1914 Minnigerode headed one of the first Red Cross hospital units (each consisting of 3 surgeons, 12 nurses, and various supplies) sent to Europe for war-relief work, and from 1914 to 1915 she served at a hospital at the Polytechnic Institute in Kiev, Russia. She then served as director of nurses at Columbia Hospital for Women in Washington, D.C. (1915–17), and she was again associated with the Red Cross from 1917 to 1919. In 1919 she was asked to make a tour of inspection of the hospitals of the U.S. Public Health Service. Her report led to the creation of a department of nurses within the service, and she was appointed superintendent. Minnigerode held that post for the rest of her life. She recruited and organized a large corps of nurses to serve in hospitals established to care for World War I veterans. Her pioneering work in that field was later taken over by the Veterans' Bureau following its establishment in August 1921. In 1925 she was awarded the Florence Nightingale Medal of the International Red Cross. By 1935 her job entailed the supervision of 650 nurses in 26 hospitals of the Public Health Service.

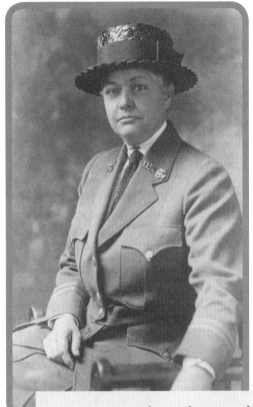

Lucy Minnigerode. Library of Congress, Washington, D.C.; neg. no. LC USZ 62 112001

MARY ADELAIDE NUTTING

(b. Nov. 1, 1858, Frost Village, District of East Canada [now Quebec, Can.]—d. Oct. 3, 1948, White Plains, N.Y., U.S.)

American nurse and educator Mary Adelaide Nutting was influential in raising the quality of higher education in nursing, hospital administration, and related fields.

Nutting grew up in Waterloo, Ontario. In 1889 she entered the first class of the new Johns Hopkins Hospital School of

Nursing in Baltimore, Maryland. After graduating in 1891 she was a head nurse in the hospital for two years and then assistant superintendent of nurses for a year. In 1894 she became superintendent of nurses and principal of the school. At that time nursing schools, even that at Johns Hopkins, were more important as sources of cheap staffing for hospitals—at a rate of from 60 to 105 hours a week from each student—than as centres of professional training. Nutting moved quickly to change the priorities in her school.

In 1895 she presented to the trustees a detailed analysis of current student nurse employment and secured approval for a new three-year curriculum, the abolition of stipends, and the institution of scholarships to needy students. She helped found the *American Journal of Nursing* in 1900. The following year she established a six-month preparation course in hygiene, elementary practical nursing, anatomy, physiology, and materia medica for entering students to prepare them for ward work. She also began a professional nursing library at Johns Hopkins, from which developed her later four-volume *History of Nursing* (1907–12, with Lavinia L. Dock). She was an early member of the American Society of Superintendents of Training Schools for Nurses of the United States and Canada (later the National League for Nursing Education; now the National League for Nursing) and twice served as president.

In 1899 an experimental program in hospital economics was established at Teachers College, Columbia University,

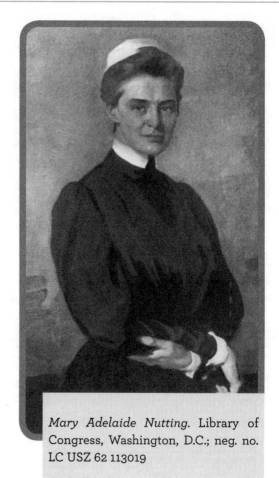

Mary Adelaide Nutting. Library of Congress, Washington, D.C.; neg. no. LC USZ 62 113019

New York City. Nutting taught part-time in the program from 1899 to 1907 and then left Johns Hopkins to become a full-time professor of institutional management at Teachers College. In 1910 she became head of the new department of nursing and health. She was the first nurse to hold either such position, and she remained at Columbia until her retirement in 1925. By that time the programs she had created in hospital administration, nursing education, public health, and other fields had brought her department international recognition. In 1934 she was named honorary president of the Florence Nightingale International Foundation, and in 1944 the National League for Nursing Education created the Mary Adelaide Nutting Medal (modeled by Malvina Hoffman) in her honour and awarded the first one to her.

MARY SEACOLE
(b. 1805, Kingston, Jamaica—d. May 14, 1881, London, Eng.)

Jamaican nurse Mary Seacole (née Mary Jane Grant) cared for British soldiers at the battlefront during the Crimean War.

Her father was a Scottish soldier and her mother a free black Jamaican woman who was skilled in traditional medicine and provided care for invalids at her boardinghouse. In 1836 Grant married Edwin Horatio Seacole, and, during their trips to the Bahamas, Haiti, and Cuba, she augmented her knowledge of local medicines and treatments. After her husband's death in 1844, she gained further nursing experience during a cholera epidemic in Panama, and, after returning to Jamaica, she cared for yellow fever victims, many of whom were British soldiers.

Seacole was in London in 1854 when reports of the lack of necessities and breakdown of nursing care for soldiers in the Crimean War began to be made public. Despite her experience, her offers to be sent to the front to help were refused, and she attributed her rejection to racial prejudice. In 1855, with the help of a relative of her husband, she went to the Crimea

as a sutler, setting up the British Hotel to sell food, supplies, and medicines to the troops. She assisted the wounded at the military hospitals and was a familiar figure at the transfer points for casualties from the front. Her remedies for cholera and dysentery were particularly valued. At the war's end she returned to England destitute and was declared bankrupt.

In 1857 her autobiography, *Wonderful Adventures of Mrs. Seacole in Many Lands*, was published and became a bestseller. A festival was held in her honour to raise funds and acknowledge her contributions, and she received decorations from France, England, and Turkey. After her death she fell into obscurity but in 2004 took first place in the 100 Great Black Britons poll in the United Kingdom.

MABEL KEATON STAUPERS
(b. Feb. 27, 1890, Barbados, West Indies—d. Nov. 29, 1989, Washington, D.C., U.S.)

Caribbean American nurse and organization executive Mabel Keaton Staupers (née Mabel Doyle) was noted for her role in eliminating segregation in the Armed Forces Nurse Corps during World War II.

Staupers immigrated to the United States with her family in 1903. In 1914 she enrolled in the Freedmen's Hospital School of Nursing (Howard University College of Nursing) in Washington, D.C., and after graduating with honours in 1917, she became a private-duty nurse. In 1920 she joined black physicians Louis T. Wright and James Wilson to establish the Booker T. Washington Sanitarium, the first hospital in Harlem to treat black Americans with tuberculosis. Staupers served as the director of nursing of the Washington Sanitarium in 1920–21 and afterward accepted a working fellowship at the Henry Phipps Institute for Tuberculosis in Philadelphia.

In 1922 Staupers returned to New York City to undertake a study of the health-care needs in Harlem. Her research led to the founding of the Harlem Committee of the New York Tuberculosis and Health Association. She became the organization's first executive secretary, a post she held for twelve years. In 1934 she was named executive secretary of the National Association of Colored Graduate Nurses (NACGN), which, owing to her early efforts, would eventually help black nurses to gain unrestricted membership in state and national nursing organizations.

Taking advantage of the high public awareness of the nursing profession during World War II, Staupers launched a campaign seeking the integration of black nurses into the Armed Forces Nurse Corps. By 1941 black nurses were admitted to the U.S. Army Nurse Corps, but a strict system of quotas hindered their full integration. The U.S. Navy continued its policy of exclusion. When the War Department began to consider a draft of nurses, Staupers enlisted the help of First Lady Eleanor Roosevelt and orchestrated a nationwide letter-writing campaign to convince President Franklin D. Roosevelt

and other political leaders of the need to recognize black nurses. Overwhelming public support of desegregation persuaded the armed forces, both Army and Navy, to wholly accept black nurses by January 1945.

Staupers' success in ending discrimination in the Armed Forces Nurse Corps buoyed her struggle for the full integration of the American Nurses Association, which was achieved in 1948. With the NACGN goal of full professional integration of black nurses having been met, the organization dissolved itself in 1951. That same year, Staupers was awarded the Spingarn Medal from the National Association for the Advancement of Colored People (NAACP). She published her autobiography, *No Time for Prejudice: A Story of the Integration of Negroes in Nursing in the United States,* in 1961.

FLORENCE WALD

(b. April 19, 1917, Bronx, N.Y., U.S.—d. Nov. 8, 2008, Branford, Conn.)

American nurse and educator Florence Wald (née Florence Sophie Schorske) reinvented the guidelines surrounding end-of-life care and was the driving force behind the building in the U.S. of a hospice system for the terminally ill, including the establishment (1974) in Branford of the first American hospice.

Wald earned three degrees from Yale University: Master of Nursing, Master of Science, and honorary Doctor of Medical Sciences, and in 1959 she was made dean of the university's school of nursing. In this role she was instrumental in introducing a more rigorous approach to the nursing curriculum and in helping nurses gain the authority to involve patients in their medical care (at the time doctors had sole authority to make medical decisions). She resigned as dean in 1966 but continued her affiliation with Yale, working as a research associate (1969–70), as a clinical associate professor (1970–80), and as a full professor (from 1980). Wald was inducted into the National Women's Hall of Fame in 1998, was honoured by the American Hospice Association with a Founder's Award, and became the recipient in 2001 of the American Academy of Nursing's Living Legend Award. At the time of her death, she was working to bring hospice care to dying prison inmates.

LILLIAN D. WALD

(b. March 10, 1867, Cincinnati, Ohio, U.S.—d. Sept. 1, 1940, Westport, Conn.)

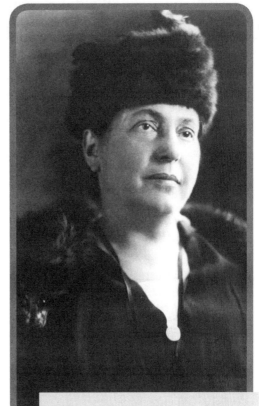

Lillian D. Wald. Library of Congress, Washington, D.C.; neg. no. LC USZ 62 34720

American nurse and social worker Lillian D. Wald founded the internationally known Henry Street Settlement in New York City (1893).

Wald grew up in her native Cincinnati, Ohio, and in Rochester, New York. She was educated in a private school, and after abandoning a plan to attend Vassar College she passed a few years enjoying an active social life. In 1889 she broke completely with that life and entered the New York Hospital Training School for Nurses, from which she graduated in 1891. For a year she worked as a nurse in the New York Juvenile Asylum. She supplemented her training in 1892–93 with courses at the Woman's Medical College. She was asked to organize a class in home nursing for the poor immigrant families of New York's Lower East Side, and in the course of that work she observed firsthand the wretched conditions within the tenement districts.

HENRY STREET SETTLEMENT

Lillian Wald founded the Henry Street Settlement in 1893. The settlement served primarily as a nursing service for immigrants. Initially comprised of several properties located on Henry Street in New York City, the settlement later expanded throughout the city's Lower East Side.

After graduating from nursing school, Wald and her colleague Mary Brewster founded the Visiting Nurse Service in 1893. That same year Wald started teaching a hygiene and home nursing class in Manhattan's Lower East Side and coined the term public health nurse *to differentiate the role of nurses who work in poor neighbourhoods. To be close to the community they served, Wald and Brewster moved into an apartment just two blocks away from the future location of the settlement. By 1894 the pair had visited 125 tenement families. When Brewster fell ill, she decided to leave the Visiting Nurse Service.*

To help finance the settlement she envisioned, Wald solicited the aid of Lower East Side German Jewish community leaders, asking them, "Have you ever seen a starving child cry?" Her appeal came to the attention of the American financier and philanthropist Jacob Schiff, who donated three Federal-style row houses he owned on Henry Street and had them converted into buildings for public use. Wald hired a staff of six nurses and moved into one of those properties.

By 1898 Henry Street Settlement had a staff of 11 full-time workers, and in 1902 it acquired three more Henry Street buildings. One included a gymnasium. The Henry Street Settlement offered English classes for new immigrants, established a savings bank, and provided vocational training, public lectures, a library, and various clubs and activities. Wald created one of New York City's first playgrounds and helped start the Outdoor Recreation League, which pushed to organize public playgrounds and parks.

Henry Street Settlement was designed as a community meeting place. Visitors were referred to simply as neighbours. Wald's mission for the settlement house was not only to provide quality services but also to be involved in social change. In 1909 Wald offered the use of the Henry Street Settlement for the National Negro Conference, which became the founding meeting for the National Association for the Advancement of Colored People (NAACP). The settlement's facilities were also used for union meetings (after the Triangle Shirtwaist Company fire); to draft child labour laws; to establish Mobilization for Youth, an urban-reform program focused on poverty and juvenile delinquency; and to help develop public housing, a government program providing affordable rental apartments to low-income, disabled, and elderly individuals.

Henry Street Settlement influenced the New York City Board of Education in 1902 to pay the salary of the first public school nurse. The New York City Board of Education and the New York City Board of Health subsequently started their own program to include 12 school nurses on the public payroll—the first such service in the world. Wald lobbied for free lunches for all children in the public school system and helped move the Board of Education to create the first Department of Special Education. By 1906 the Henry Street Settlement had a team of 27 nurses aiding the Lower East Side. By 1914 that number had grown to more than 100.

In 1908 Henry Street Settlement opened two summer camps: Camp Henry for boys and Echo Hill Farm for girls. The Neighborhood Playhouse (later renamed the Harry De Jur Playhouse) opened in 1915. It was used for Henry Street Settlement art programs. The Henry Street Music School was opened in 1927.

At the time of Wald's death in 1940, nearly 300 nurses worked out of 20 branches of the Henry Street Settlement around New York City. In 1989 the three original Henry Street buildings were designated a national historic landmark. They are America's oldest existing settlement house.

In the autumn of 1893, with Mary M. Brewster, Wald left medical school, moved to the neighbourhood, and offered her services as a visiting nurse. Two years later, with aid from banker-philanthropist Jacob H. Schiff and others, she took larger accommodations and opened the Nurse's Settlement. As the number of nurses attached to the settlement grew (from the original 2 in 1893 to 92 in 1913 and to more than 250 by 1929), services were expanded to include nurses' training, educational programs for the community, and youth clubs. Within a few years the Henry Street establishment had become a neighbourhood centre, the Henry Street Settlement.

Over the years the settlement was a powerful source of innovation in the social settlement movement and in the broader field of social work generally. The Neighborhood Playhouse was opened in connection with the settlement in 1915 through the benefaction of Irene Lewisohn. Residents at Henry Street included at various times social reformer Florence Kelley, economist Adolf A. Berle, Jr., labour leader Sidney Hillman, and Henry Morgenthau, Jr., U.S. secretary of the Treasury under President Franklin D. Roosevelt. Wald exerted considerable influence beyond Henry Street as well. In 1902, at her initiative, nursing service was experimentally extended to a local public school, and soon the municipal board of health instituted a citywide public school nursing program, the first such program in the world. The organization of nursing programs by insurance companies for their industrial policyholders (pioneered by the Metropolitan Life Insurance Company in 1909) and of the district nursing service of the Red Cross (begun in 1912 and later called Town and Country Nursing Service) were both at her suggestion.

In 1912 Wald's role as founder of an entirely new profession was formally acknowledged when she helped found and became first president of the National Organization for Public Health Nursing. She also worked to establish educational, recreational, and social programs in underprivileged neighbourhoods. In 1912 Congress established the U.S. Children's Bureau (headed by Julia Lathrop), also in no small part owing to Wald's suggestion, and in that year she was awarded the gold medal of the National Institute of Social Sciences.

Wald was active in other areas of reform, particularly with the National Child Labor Committee, which she and Florence Kelley helped found in 1903, the national Women's Trade Union League, and the American Union Against Militarism, which she, Kelley, and Jane Addams helped organize in 1914 and of which she was elected president. During World War I she headed the committee on home nursing of the Council of National Defense. She led the Nurses' Emergency Council in the influenza epidemic of 1918–19. Later she founded the League of Free Nations, a forerunner of the Foreign Policy Association. She wrote two autobiographical books, *The House on Henry Street* (1915) and *Windows on Henry Street* (1934). In 1933 ill health forced her to resign as head worker of Henry Street, and she settled in Westport, Connecticut.

CHAPTER 9

PIONEERS OF MODERN MEDICINE

Countless physicians and medical researchers have contributed to the advance of modern medicine, far more individuals than can be covered in any single work. Furthermore, their contributions are so diverse and varied in nature that characterizing these individuals in any systematic way is nearly impossible—with the exception that all can be considered pioneers of modern medicine. The names of many of these individuals—Mayo, Apgar, Osler—are familiar and well known, particularly within the scientific and medical communities.

SIR THOMAS CLIFFORD ALLBUTT

(b. July 20, 1836, Dewsbury, Yorkshire, Eng.—d. Feb. 22, 1925, Cambridge, Cambridgeshire)

English physician Sir Thomas Clifford Allbutt invented the short clinical thermometer. His investigations also led to the improved treatment of arterial diseases.

During a 28-year practice in Leeds, Allbutt made valuable clinical studies, primarily of arterial and nervous disorders. In 1866 he introduced the modern clinical thermometer, a welcome alternative to the foot-long instrument that required 20 minutes to register a patient's temperature. In 1871 he published a monograph outlining use of the ophthalmoscope (used to inspect the interior of the eye) as a diagnostic instrument. In 1892 Allbutt became regius professor of physic at the University of Cambridge, where he spent the rest of his career. Continuing his previous work, he postulated that the painful heart condition angina pectoris originates in the aorta (1894).

Allbutt was also a noted medical historian. Two of his most important publications were *Diseases of the Arteries, Including Angina Pectoris* (1915) and *Greek Medicine in Rome* (1921). He also edited *A System of Medicine*, 8 vol. (1896–99). He was knighted in 1907.

ELIZABETH GARRETT ANDERSON
(b. June 9, 1836, Aldeburgh, Suffolk, Eng.—d. Dec. 17, 1917, Aldeburgh)

English physician Elizabeth Garrett Anderson advocated the admission of

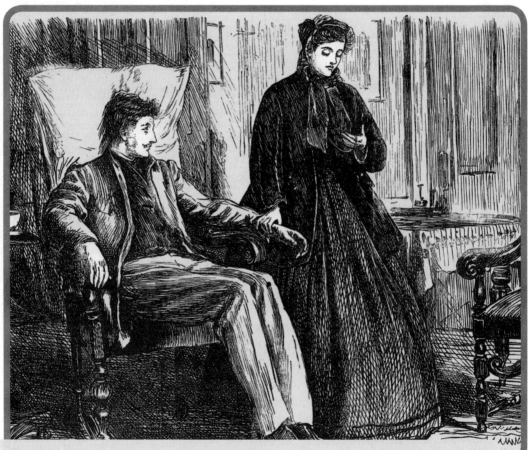

Elizabeth Garrett Anderson with a patient, 19th-century illustration. Photos.com/ Jupiterimages

women to professional education, especially in medicine.

Refused admission to medical schools, Anderson began in 1860 to study privately with accredited physicians and in London hospitals and was licensed to practice in 1865 by the Society of Apothecaries. She was appointed (1866) general medical attendant to the Marylebone Dispensary, later the New Hospital for Women, where she worked to create a medical school for women. In 1918 the hospital was renamed Elizabeth Garrett Anderson Hospital in her honour. Anderson received the M.D. degree from the University of Paris in 1870, and in 1908 she became the first woman mayor of Aldeburgh.

VIRGINIA APGAR

(b. June 7, 1909, Westfield, N.J., U.S.—d. Aug. 7, 1974, New York, N.Y.)

American physician, anesthesiologist, and medical researcher Virginia Apgar developed the Apgar Score System, a method of evaluating an infant shortly after birth to assess its well-being and to determine if any immediate medical intervention is required.

Apgar graduated from Mount Holyoke College in 1929 and from the Columbia University College of Physicians and Surgeons in 1933. After an internship at Presbyterian Hospital, New York City, she held residencies in the relatively new specialty of anesthesiology at the University of Wisconsin and then at Bellevue Hospital, New York City, in 1935–37. In 1937 she became the first female board-certified anesthesiologist. The first professor of anesthesiology at the College of Physicians and Surgeons (1949–59), she was also the first female physician to attain the rank of full professor there. Additionally, from 1938 she was director of the department of anesthesiology at Columbia-Presbyterian Medical Center.

An interest in obstetric procedure, and particularly in the treatment of the newborn, led her to develop a simple system for quickly evaluating the condition and viability of newly delivered infants. As finally presented in 1952, the Apgar Score System relies on five simple observations to be made by delivery room personnel (nurses or interns) of the infant within one minute of birth and—depending on the results of the first observation—periodically thereafter. The Apgar Score System soon came into general use throughout the United States and was adopted by several other countries.

In 1959 Apgar left Columbia and took a degree in public health from Johns Hopkins University. She headed the division of congenital malformations at the National Foundation-March of Dimes from 1959–67. She was promoted to director of basic research at the National Foundation (1967–72), and she later became senior vice president for medical affairs (1973–74). She cowrote the book *Is My Baby All Right?* (1972) with Joan Beck.

APGAR SCORE SYSTEM

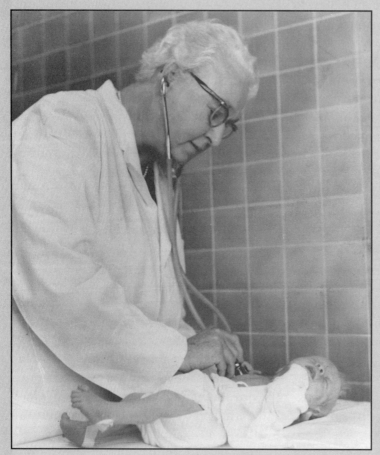

Virginia Apgar examining a baby, 1966. Al Ravenna—World Journal Tribune/Library of Congress, Washington, D.C. (dig. id. cph 3c31540)

The Apgar Score System is a medical rating procedure developed in 1952 by Dr. Virginia Apgar to evaluate the condition of newborn infants and to identify those that require life-sustaining medical assistance, such as resuscitation. The Apgar score is a qualitative measurement of a newborn's success in adapting to the environment outside the uterus.

A newborn infant is evaluated one minute and five minutes after birth. Five signs are assessed: heart rate, respiratory effort, muscle tone, reflex irritability, and skin colour. Medical students memorize these signs by using the mnemonic of Apgar's name: appearance, pulse, grimace, activity, and respiration. A score of 0, 1, or 2 is assigned to each component. Usually, the higher the total score, with 10 being the maximum, the better the infant's condition. If the infant's total score is less than 7, it is reevaluated every 5 minutes until 20 minutes have passed or until two successive scores of 7 or greater are obtained.

According to some researchers, the one- and five-minute Apgar scores are of limited use in predicting the degree of asphyxia (lack of oxygen or excess of carbon dioxide) or the consequences of any neurological involvement. Apgar scores taken at 10 or 15 minutes may be more successful indicators of an infant's later neurological deficit.

OSWALD AVERY

(b. Oct. 21, 1877, Halifax, N.S., Can.—d. Feb. 20, 1955, Nashville, Tenn., U.S.)

Canadian-born American bacteriologist Oswald Avery helped ascertain that DNA is the substance responsible for heredity, thus laying the foundation for the new science of molecular genetics. His work also contributed to the understanding of the chemistry of immunological processes.

Avery received a medical degree from Columbia University College of Physicians and Surgeons in New York City in 1904. After a few years in clinical practice, he joined the Hoagland Laboratory in Brooklyn and turned his attention to bacteriological research. In 1913 he joined the staff of the Rockefeller Institute Hospital in New York City, where he began studying the bacterium responsible for lobar pneumonia, Streptococcus pneumoniae, called the pneumococcus. Avery and colleagues isolated a substance in the blood and urine of infected persons that was produced by this bacterium. They identified the substance as a complex carbohydrate called a polysaccharide, which makes up the capsular envelope of the pneumococcus. Based on the recognition that the polysaccharide composition of capsular envelopes can vary, Avery helped classify pneumococci into different types. Avery also found that the polysaccharide could stimulate an immune response—specifically, the production

of antibodies—and was the first to demonstrate that a substance other than a protein could do so. The evidence that the polysaccharide composition of a bacterium influences its virulence (ability to cause disease) and its immunological specificity showed that these characteristics can be analyzed biochemically, thus contributing to the development of immunochemistry.

In 1932 Avery turned his attention to an experiment carried out by a British microbiologist named Frederick Griffith. Griffith worked with two strains of S. pneumoniae—one encircled by a polysaccharide capsule that was virulent, and another that lacked a capsule and was nonvirulent. Griffith's results showed that the virulent strain could somehow convert, or transform, the nonvirulent strain into an agent of disease. Furthermore, the transformation was heritable—i.e., able to be passed on to succeeding generations of bacteria. Avery, along with many other scientists, set out to determine the chemical nature of the substance that allowed transformation to occur. In 1944 he and his colleagues Maclyn McCarty and Colin MacLeod reported that the transforming substance—the genetic material of the cell—was DNA. This result was met initially with skepticism, as many scientists believed that proteins would prove to be the repository of hereditary information. Eventually, however, the role of DNA was proved, and Avery's contribution to genetics was recognized.

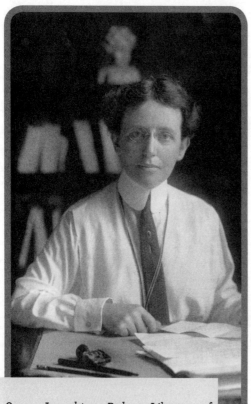

Sara Josephine Baker. Library of Congress, Washington, D.C.; neg. no. LC USZ 62 058326

SARA JOSEPHINE BAKER

(b. Nov. 15, 1873, Poughkeepsie, N.Y., U.S.—d. Feb. 22, 1945, New York, N.Y.),

American physician Sara Josephine Baker contributed significantly to public health and child welfare in the United States.

Baker prepared at private schools for Vassar College, but the death of her father put that school out of reach. She decided to study medicine and after a year of private preparation entered the Women's Medical College of the New York Infirmary in New York City. After graduating in 1898 she interned at the New England Hospital for Women and Children and then entered private practice in New York City.

In 1901 Baker was appointed a medical inspector for the city health department, and in 1907 she became assistant to the commissioner of health. In that post she aided in the apprehension of "Typhoid Mary" Mallon. More importantly, however, she developed from the rudimentary program of inspection for infectious diseases a comprehensive approach to preventive health care for children. In the summer of 1908 she was allowed to test her plan in a slum district on the East Side. A team of 30 nurses under her direction sought out every infant in the district, taught simple hygiene—ventilation, bathing, light clothing, breast-feeding—to the mothers, and made follow-up visits. At the end of the summer the district had recorded 1,200 fewer cases of infant mortality than the previous summer.

In August 1908 the Division of Child Hygiene was established in the health department and Baker was named director. The division (later raised to bureau) was the first government agency in the world devoted to child health. There Baker evolved a broad program including strict examination and licensing of midwives (and from 1911 free instruction at Bellevue Hospital), appointment of school nurses and doctors, compulsory use of silver nitrate drops in the eyes of all newborns, inspection of schoolchildren for infectious diseases, and numerous methods of distributing information on health and hygiene among the poor.

To deal with the inescapable problem faced by working mothers, Baker organized "Little Mothers' Leagues" to provide training to young girls required to care for infants. In 1911 she organized and became president of the Babies Welfare Association; the next year it was reorganized as the Children's Welfare Federation of New York, of which she was president until 1914 and chairman of the executive committee in 1914–17. As a result of her division's work, the infant mortality rate in New York City fell from 144 per 1,000 live births in 1908 to 88 in 1918 and 66 in 1923. By that time the division's health stations were caring for some 60,000 babies a year—half those born in the city. From 1916 to 1930 she lectured on child hygiene at the New York University-Bellevue Hospital Medical School, and in 1917 she was the first woman to receive from it a doctorate in public health. For 16 years, from its organization in 1912, she was a staff consultant to the federal Children's Bureau. After her retirement from the Bureau of Child Hygiene in 1923, she became a consultant to the Children's Bureau and a representative on child health issues to the League of Nations. In addition to articles in popular and professional journals, Baker published *Healthy Babies*, *Healthy Children*, and *Healthy Mothers* (all 1920), *The Growing Child* (1923), *Child Hygiene* (1925), and an autobiography, *Fighting for Life* (1939).

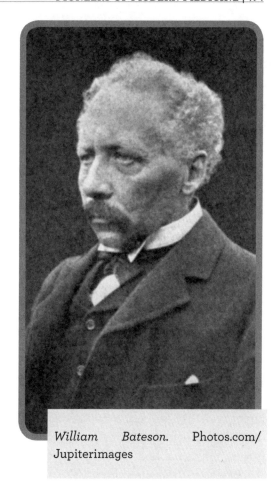

William Bateson. Photos.com/ Jupiterimages

WILLIAM BATESON
(b. Aug. 8, 1861, Whitby, Yorkshire, Eng.—d. Feb. 8, 1926, London)

English biologist William Bateson founded and named the science of genetics and was known for his experiments that provided evidence basic to the modern understanding of heredity. A dedicated evolutionist, he cited embryo studies to support his contention in 1885 that chordates evolved from primitive echinoderms, a view now widely accepted. In 1894 he published his conclusion (*Materials for the Study of Variation*) that evolution could not occur through a continuous variation of species, since distinct features often appeared or disappeared suddenly in plants and animals. Realizing that discontinuous variation could be understood only after something was known about the inheritance of traits, Bateson began work on the experimental breeding of plants and animals.

In 1900, he discovered an article, "Experiments with Plant Hybrids," written by Gregor Mendel, an Austrian monk, 34 years earlier. The paper, found in the same year by Hugo de Vries, Carl Correns, and Erich Tschermak von Seysenegg, dealt with the appearance of certain features in successive generations of garden peas. Bateson noted that his breeding results were explained perfectly by Mendel's paper and that the monk had succinctly described the transmission of elements governing heritable traits in his plants.

Bateson translated Mendel's paper into English and during the next 10 years became Mendel's champion in England, corroborating his principles experimentally. He published, with Reginald Punnett, the results of a series of breeding experiments (1905–08) that not only extended Mendel's principles to animals (poultry) but showed also that certain features were consistently inherited together, apparently counter to Mendel's findings. This phenomenon, which came to be termed linkage, is now known to be the result of the occurrence of genes located in close proximity on the same chromosome. Bateson's experiments also demonstrated a dependence of certain characters on two or more genes. Unfortunately, he misinterpreted his results, refusing to accept the interpretation of linkage advanced by the geneticist Thomas Hunt Morgan. In fact, he opposed Morgan's entire chromosome theory, advocating his own vibratory theory of inheritance, founded on laws of force and motion, a concept that found little acceptance among other scientists.

Bateson became, at the University of Cambridge, the first British professor of genetics (1908). He left this chair in 1910 to spend the rest of his life directing the John Innes Horticultural Institution at Merton, South London (later moved to Norwich), transforming it into a centre for genetic research. His books include *Mendel's Principles of Heredity* (1902, 2nd edition published in 1909) and *Problems of Genetics* (1913).

ALEXANDER GORDON BEARN
(b. March 29, 1923, Cheam, Surrey, Eng.—d. May 15, 2009, Philadelphia, Pa., U.S.)

British-born American physician and geneticist Alexander Gordon Bearn discovered the hereditary nature of Wilson disease and established the basis for diagnostic tests and novel forms of treatment for the disease. Bearn's work, which provided an important model for the identification, diagnosis, and treatment of other genetic diseases, served to bridge the gap between genetics and medicine that existed in the 1950s.

Bearn received a Bachelor of Medicine degree in 1946 from King's College School of Medicine and Dentistry, University of London. He continued his doctoral studies there, eventually receiving a Doctorate of Medicine degree in 1950. The following year he left England to take a position as an assistant professor at the Rockefeller Institute for Medical Research (now Rockefeller University) in New York City. There Bearn became interested in the genetic mutations underlying rare metabolic diseases and eventually narrowed his research, focusing on Wilson disease. Although diseases caused by hereditary defects had been described in the early 20th century, they were not understood well enough to facilitate their diagnosis or to encourage the development of improved treatments. Thus, when Bearn began investigating Wilson disease, genetics was of little consequence to medicine. In 1957 Bearn established one of the first human genetics laboratories in the United States at Rockefeller, and in 1964 he became a professor of medicine there.

Wilson disease was described as progressive lenticular degeneration in 1912 by American-born British neurologist Samuel A.K. Wilson. Wilson's autopsies of affected patients revealed cirrhosis of the liver and degeneration of the lenticular nucleus, a part of the brain located within the basal ganglia. In the following decades, it was found that the liver and brain served as sites for the accumulation of copper, which was discovered to be the underlying pathological feature of the disease. Although Wilson and others found that the disease occurred within families, it was not recognized as a hereditary condition. In fact, it was not until the 1950s, when Bearn studied families affected by Wilson disease and found that it was inherited in an autosomal recessive fashion, that the hereditary nature of the condition was realized. The recessive inheritance of Wilson disease meant that two copies (one from each parent) of the abnormal gene were required to cause the disease.

Bearn proposed that the specific genetic defect of Wilson disease, which was unknown then, somehow altered the transport of copper into and out of cells. Bearn suggested that a serum protein called ceruloplasmin, which transports copper through the blood and is present in abnormally low levels in Wilson disease patients, could be used as a diagnostic measure for the disease. In addition, decreased serum levels and decreased urinary excretion of copper also could serve as measures for diagnosis. For the treatment of Wilson disease, Bearn promoted the use of penicillamine, a chelating agent that lowers tissue concentrations of copper by drawing the element out of cells and facilitating its excretion in the urine. Bearn also encouraged patients to avoid eating foods that are high in copper.

In 1966 Bearn was appointed chairman of the department of medicine at Cornell University Medical College. He subsequently established a human genetics laboratory there and became physician in chief at New York Hospital (now New York–Presbyterian Hospital). While at Cornell, Bearn helped initiate a joint M.D./Ph.D. program between Cornell and Rockefeller. In 1970 Bearn joined Rockefeller's board of trustees, and the following year he became president of the American Society of Human Genetics. In 1972 he was elected a member of the American Philosophical Society, a prestigious organization founded by Benjamin Franklin in 1743. Bearn later served as vice president (1990–96) and as executive officer (1997–2002) of the society and was elected a member of the National Academy of Science. From 1979 to 1988 Bearn served as senior vice president for medical and scientific affairs for the pharmaceutical company Merck & Co., Inc.

Following his retirement from Cornell in 1988, Bearn wrote *Sir Archibald Garrod and the Individuality of Man* (1993), which explores the life and discoveries of Garrod, who was a British physician and geneticist known for his investigations into inherited metabolic diseases in the early 1900s. Bearn later wrote two other biographies, *Sir Clifford Allbutt: Scholar and Physician* (2007) and *Sir Francis Richard Fraser: A Canny Scot Shapes British Medicine* (2008).

ELIZABETH BLACKWELL

(b. Feb. 3, 1821, Counterslip, Bristol, Gloucestershire, Eng.—d. May 31, 1910, Hastings, Sussex)

English-born physician Elizabeth Blackwell is considered the first woman doctor of medicine in modern times.

Elizabeth Blackwell was of a large, prosperous, and cultured family and was well educated by private tutors. Financial reverses and the family's liberal social and religious views prompted them to immigrate to the United States in the summer of 1832. Soon after taking up residence in New York, her father, Samuel Blackwell, became active in abolitionist activities. The Blackwells moved to Jersey City, New Jersey, in 1835 and to Cincinnati, Ohio, in 1838. Soon afterward Samuel Blackwell's death left the family in poverty, and Elizabeth and two sisters opened a private school. Later Elizabeth taught school in Henderson, Kentucky, and in 1845–47 in North and South Carolina.

During the latter period Elizabeth Blackwell undertook the study of medicine privately with sympathetic physicians, and in 1847 she began seeking admission to a medical school. All the leading schools rejected her application, but she was at length admitted, almost by fluke, to Geneva Medical College (a forerunner of Hobart College) in Geneva, New York. Her months there were extremely difficult. Townspeople and much of the male student body ostracized and harassed her, and she was at first even barred from classroom demonstration. She persevered, however, and in January 1849, ranked first in her class, she became the first woman in the United States to graduate from medical school and the first modern-day woman doctor of medicine.

In April, having become a naturalized U.S. citizen, Blackwell traveled to

England to seek further training, and in May she went on to Paris, where in June she entered the midwives' course at La Maternité. While there she contracted an infectious eye disease that left her blind in one eye and forced her to abandon hope of becoming a surgeon. In October 1850 she returned to England and worked at St. Bartholomew's Hospital under Dr. (later Sir) James Paget. In the summer of 1851 she returned to New York, where she was refused posts in the city's hospitals and dispensaries and was even unable to rent private consulting quarters. Her private practice was very slow to develop, and in the meantime she wrote a series of lectures, published in 1852 as *The Laws of Life, with Special Reference to the Physical Education of Girls.*

In 1853 Blackwell opened a small dispensary in a slum district. Within a few years she was joined by her younger sister, Dr. Emily Blackwell, and by Dr. Marie E. Zakrzewska, and in May 1857 the dispensary, greatly enlarged, was incorporated as the New York Infirmary for Women and Children. In January 1859, during a year-long lecture tour of Great Britain, she became the first woman to have her name placed on the British medical register. At the outbreak of the American Civil War in 1861, she helped organize the Woman's Central Association of Relief and the U.S. Sanitary Commission and worked mainly through the former to select and train nurses for war service.

In November 1868 a plan long in the perfecting, developed in large part in consultation with Florence Nightingale in England, bore fruit in the opening of the Woman's Medical College at the infirmary. Elizabeth Blackwell set very high standards for admission, academic and clinical training, and certification for the school, which continued in operation for 31 years; she herself occupied the chair of hygiene. In 1869 Blackwell moved permanently to England. She established a successful private practice, helped organize the National Health Society in 1871, and in 1875 was appointed professor of gynecology at the London School of Medicine for Women. She retained the latter position until 1907, when an injury forced her to retire. Among her other writings are *The Religion of Health* (1871), *Counsel to Parents on the Moral Education of Their Children* (1878), *The Human Element in Sex* (1884), her autobiographical *Pioneer Work in Opening the Medical Profession to Women* (1895), and *Essays in Medical Sociology* (1902).

BARUCH S. BLUMBERG
(b. July 28, 1925, New York, N.Y., U.S.)

American research physician Baruch S. Blumberg was known for his discovery of an antigen that provokes antibody response against hepatitis B. This finding led to the development by other researchers of a successful vaccine against the disease. He shared the Nobel Prize in Physiology or Medicine in 1976 with D. Carleton Gajdusek for their work on the origins and spread of infectious viral diseases.

Blumberg received his M.D. degree from Columbia University's College of Physicians and Surgeons and his Ph.D. degree in biochemistry from Oxford University in 1957. In 1960 he became chief of the Geographic Medicine and Genetics Section of the U.S. National Institutes for Health, in Maryland. In 1964 he was appointed associate director for clinical research at the Institute for Cancer Research (later named the Fox Chase Cancer Center) in Philadelphia, and in 1977 he became professor of medicine, human genetics, and anthropology at the University of Pennsylvania. In 1989 he returned to Oxford to become master of Balliol College, a position that he held until 1994. Upon his return to the United States, he resumed his post at the Fox Chase Cancer Center, gaining the title Distinguished Scientist, and continued to teach as professor of medicine and anthropology at the University of Pennsylvania. In May 1999 Blumberg was appointed director of the National Aeronautics and Space Administration (NASA) Astrobiology Institute. He held several different positions while at NASA, where he remained until 2004. The following year he was elected president of the American Philosophical Society.

In the early 1960s Blumberg was examining blood samples from widely diverse populations in an attempt to determine why the members of different ethnic and national groups vary widely in their responses and susceptibility to disease. In 1963 he discovered in the blood serum of an Australian aborigine an antigen that he later (1967) determined to be part of a virus that causes hepatitis B, the most severe form of hepatitis. The discovery of this so-called Australian antigen, which causes the body to produce antibody responses to the virus, made it possible to screen blood donors for possible hepatitis B transmission. Further research indicated that the body's development of antibody against the Australian antigen was protective against further infection with the virus itself. In 1982 a safe and effective vaccine utilizing Australian antigen was made commercially available in the United States.

EMELINE HORTON CLEVELAND

(b. Sept. 22, 1829, Ashford, Conn., U.S.—d. Dec. 8, 1878, Philadelphia, Pa.)

American physician and college professor Emeline Horton Cleveland (née Emeline Horton) was a strong proponent of professional opportunity and education for women in medicine.

Emeline Horton grew up in Madison county, New York. She worked as a teacher until she could afford to enroll at Oberlin (Ohio) College, from which she graduated in 1853. She then entered the Female (later Woman's) Medical College of Pennsylvania in Philadelphia and took her M.D. degree in 1855. While working toward her medical degree she married the Reverend Giles B. Cleveland. Her husband's ill health ended their plan to undertake missionary work, and, after a year of private practice, Cleveland became a demonstrator of anatomy at the Female Medical College. She soon was named professor of anatomy and histology. In 1860–61, with the support of Ann Preston, a doctor at the college, Cleveland took advanced training in obstetrics at the school of the Maternité hospital in Paris. Upon her return to Philadelphia, she became chief resident at the rechartered Woman's Medical College, a post she held until 1868. From 1862 she also taught obstetrics and diseases of women and children and carried on an extensive private practice.

Cleveland's professional reputation was unsurpassed among women physicians. On several occasions she was consulted by male colleagues, and she eventually was admitted to membership in several all-male local medical societies. Her work at the college, where she had early established training courses for nurses and for nurse's aides (the latter a pioneering venture), was capped by her tenure as dean, succeeding Preston, in 1872–74. In 1875, in what was apparently the earliest recorded instance of major surgery performed by a woman, she performed the first of several ovariotomies. In 1878 she was appointed gynecologist to the department for the insane at Pennsylvania Hospital, but she died late that year.

MARY PUTNAM JACOBI

(b. Aug. 31, 1842, London, Eng.—d. June 10, 1906, New York, N.Y., U.S.)

American physician, writer, and suffragist Mary Putnam Jacobi (née Mary Corinna Putnam) is considered to have been the foremost woman doctor of her era.

Mary Putnam was the daughter of George Palmer Putnam, founder of the publishing firm of G.P. Putnam's Sons, and was an elder sister of Herbert Putnam, later librarian of Congress. The family returned from England in 1848, and Mary grew up in Staten Island, Yonkers, and Morrisania, New York. Her scientific bent determined her on a medical career, but in 1860, before she was 18, she had a story published in *The Atlantic Monthly*. She graduated from the New York College of Pharmacy in 1863 and from the Female (later Woman's) Medical College of Pennsylvania in 1864.

After working for a few months at the New England Hospital for Women and Children in Boston, Putnam decided in 1866 to seek further training in Paris. There she attended clinics, lectures, and a class at the École Pratique until she decided to seek admission to the École de Médecine. Her persistence finally secured a directive from the minister of education forcing the faculty to admit her in 1868. Her course was a distinguished one, and she graduated in 1871 with a prizewinning thesis. During her stay in Paris she contributed letters, articles, and stories to the *Medical Record*, *Putnam's Magazine*, the *New York Evening Post*, and *Scribner's Monthly*.

In the fall of 1871 Putnam returned to New York City, opened a practice, and began teaching at Dr. Elizabeth Blackwell's Woman's Medical College of the New York Infirmary for Women and Children. The quality of her own education had highlighted for her the meagreness of that available to most women aiming for a medical career, and in 1872 she organized the Association for the Advancement of the Medical Education of Women (later the Women's Medical Association of New York City) to begin redressing that shortcoming; she was president of the association from 1874 to 1903. In 1873 she married Dr. Abraham Jacobi, generally considered the founder of pediatrics in America. In the same year, Mary Jacobi began a children's dispensary service at Mount Sinai Hospital. From 1882 to 1885 she lectured on diseases of children at the New York Post-Graduate Medical School. She opened a small children's ward at the New York Infirmary in 1886. She resigned her professorship at the Woman's Medical College in 1889 but continued to be a force for improved education for women. From 1893 she was visiting physician at St. Mark's Hospital. In addition to clinical work and teaching, she found time for writing as well.

Jacobi's bibliography runs to more than a hundred titles, mainly in pathology, neurology, pediatrics, and medical education, and one of her essays won the 1876 Boylston Prize from Harvard. Her books include *The Value of Life* (1879), *Essays on Hysteria, Brain-Tumor, and Some Other Cases of Nervous Disease* (1888), *Physiological Notes on Primary Education and the Study of Language* (1889), and *"Common Sense" Applied to Woman Suffrage* (1894). While she did

little original research, her contribution to the status of women within the medical profession was incalculable. She also took an interest in social causes. She helped found the Working Women's Society (from 1890 the New York Consumers' League) and the League for Political Education.

MAYO FAMILY

(b. May 31, 1819, near Manchester, Eng.—d. March 6, 1911, Rochester, Minn., U.S.), (b. June 29, 1861, Le Sueur, Minn.—d. July 28, 1939, Rochester), (b. July 19, 1865, Rochester—d. May 26, 1939, Chicago, Ill.), (b. July 28, 1898, Rochester—d. July 28, 1968, Rochester)

William Worrall Mayo, William James Mayo, Charles Horace Mayo, and Charles William Mayo, respectively, otherwise known as the Mayo family, were arguably the most famous physicians in the United States. Three generations of the Mayo family established at Rochester, Minn., the world-renowned nonprofit Mayo Clinic and the Mayo Foundation for Medical Education and Research, which are dedicated to diagnosing and treating nearly every known illness.

William Worrall Mayo was the father of the doctors Mayo who developed a large-scale practice of medicine. Mayo studied chemistry at Owens College in Manchester and, after immigrating to the United States in 1845, learned medicine from a private physician in Lafayette, Ind., subsequently receiving degrees from Indiana Medical College,

La Porte, and the University of Missouri, Columbia. In 1863 he moved to Rochester, where he soon had an extensive surgical practice. After taking care of the casualties of a disastrous tornado in Rochester, with the assistance of the Sisters of St. Francis, Mayo, his two sons, and the sisters planned to erect a new hospital. St. Mary's Hospital was opened on Oct. 1, 1889, and Mayo and his two sons became responsible for care of the patients. After the father retired, the work at the hospital was continued by his sons.

William James Mayo was the eldest son of William Worrall Mayo. He received his M.D. degree in 1883 from the University of Michigan, Ann Arbor, and then engaged at Rochester in the private practice of medicine and surgery with his father and later with his younger brother Charles Horace Mayo. Though William J. Mayo became the administrator in the practice, no important decisions were made without the full agreement of both brothers. He and his brother performed all the surgeries at St. Mary's Hospital until about 1905. From this surgical partnership of the two brothers evolved the cooperative group clinic, later known as the Mayo Clinic. William James Mayo, who became a specialist in surgery of the abdomen, pelvis, and kidney, remained active in surgery at the clinic until 1928 and in administration until 1933.

Charles Horace Mayo, the younger son of William Worrall Mayo, was characterized as a "surgical wonder." He received an M.D. degree from the Chicago Medical College (later part of Northwestern University Medical School) in 1888 and in the same year began private practice of surgery with his father and brother.

Charles Mayo had the ability to work in all surgical fields; he originated modern procedures in goitre surgery and in neurosurgery; he performed highly successful operations for cataract of the eye and originated procedures for several orthopedic operations. In 1930 he retired from surgery at the clinic and three years later from administration. He was professor of surgery at the University of Minnesota Medical School from 1919 to 1936 and at the University of Minnesota Graduate School from 1915 to 1936. In regard to his brother, William J. Mayo said, "Charlie has...an intuitive mind, from his knowledge of physiology and anatomy and his understanding of the personality of the patient." At one time he was a member of the advisory board of *Encyclopædia Britannica*. With his brother, he alternated as chief consultant for all surgical services in the U.S. Army during World War I, serving with the rank of colonel. After the war, each brother was commissioned a brigadier general in the medical-corps reserve.

Charles William Mayo was the son of Charles Horace. He was a skilled surgeon and member of the board of governors of the Mayo Clinic, chairman of the Mayo Association, and a member (chairman 1961–67) of the board of regents of the University of Minnesota. He is noted for a speech he gave in 1953 as a member of the United States delegation at the United Nations.

The clinic began to grow in size in the early 1900s, when many young physicians began to apply for positions as interns and assistants. At the same time, outstanding scientists in basic medical subjects were added to the clinic's training and research programs. In 1919 the Mayo brothers transferred property and capital to the Mayo Properties Association, later called the Mayo Foundation, a charitable and educational corporation having a perpetual charter. About 1900 the Mayo Clinic was changed from a partnership to a voluntary association of physicians and specialists in allied fields.

In 1915 the Mayo brothers gave $1.5 million to the University of Minnesota to establish the Mayo Foundation for Medical Education and Research at Rochester in connection with the clinic. The foundation, which is part of the University of Minnesota Graduate School, offers graduate training in medicine and related subjects.

In 1986 the Mayo Clinic merged with the nearby St. Mary's Hospital and Rochester Methodist Hospital. The Mayo Foundation also began a national expansion program that year, opening the Mayo Clinic Jacksonville in Florida; the Mayo Clinic Scottsdale in Arizona opened in 1987. In 1992 the Mayo Foundation launched the Mayo Health System, a network of clinics, hospitals, and health-care facilities (including nursing homes) serving communities in Iowa, Minnesota, and Wisconsin.

In the early 21st century the Mayo Clinic's three sites employed more than 3,300 physicians, researchers, and scientists and more than 46,000 allied health staff and treated more than 500,000 patients annually. The clinic produces several publications, including *Mayo Magazine*.

MENNINGER FAMILY
(b. July 11, 1862, Tell City, Ind., U.S.—d. Nov. 28, 1953, Topeka, Kan.), (b. July 22, 1893, Topeka—d. July 18, 1990, Topeka), (b. Oct. 15, 1899, Topeka—d. Sept. 6, 1966, Topeka)

Charles Frederick Menninger, Karl Augustus Menninger, and William Claire Menninger, respectively, were American physicians who pioneered methods of psychiatric treatment in the 20th century.

Charles Frederick Menninger began practicing general medicine in Topeka in 1889 and became convinced of the benefit of group medical practice after visiting the Mayo Clinic in Rochester, Minnesota, in 1908. Menninger was joined in practice by his son Karl Augustus Menninger, who received his medical degree from Harvard Medical School in 1917 and who spent two years working under Ernest Southard at the Boston Psychopathic Hospital. In 1919 the two Menningers established the Menninger Diagnostic Clinic in Topeka for the group practice of general medicine. Karl Menninger's strong interest in psychiatry and the Topeka area's lack of hospital care for the mentally ill led him to treat psychiatric patients as well. In 1924 Charles Menninger's youngest son, William

Claire Menninger, received his M.D. from Cornell University Medical College and served his internship at Bellevue Hospital in New York City. The following year, he joined the family practice.

In 1925 the family established the Menninger Sanitarium and Psychopathic Hospital, a facility designed to apply group medical practice to psychiatric patients. In this and other facilities that followed, the Menningers linked two concepts: (1) the psychoanalytic understanding of behaviour as applied to the treatment of hospitalized patients and (2) the use of the social environment of the hospital as an adjunct to therapy. Thus, in the Menningers' attempt to merge the psychiatric treatment of their patients with the local environment, all members of the clinic's staff—nurses, therapists, orderlies, and even housekeepers—became an attentive and helpful part of the patients' milieu. From the onset, psychiatric research was an important part of the Menningers' total approach. The Menningers' care and treatment of the mentally ill began to draw scientists interested in their ideas and eager to study at the hospital. In 1926 the Menningers opened the Southard School for mentally retarded children, and in a matter of years they were accepting children with all types of mental disorders.

The Menningers' philosophy that psychiatry is a legitimate science and that the difference between a "normal" individual and a person with a mental illness is but a matter of degree was expounded in Karl Menninger's first book, *The Human Mind*

(1930), which became a best seller. In 1931 the Menninger Sanitarium became the first institution to gain approval as a training facility for nurses specializing in psychiatric care, and in 1933 it opened a neuropsychiatric residency program for physicians.

The formation of the Menninger Foundation in 1941 not only fulfilled the family's goal of combining medical practice, research, and education on an international level but also marked the beginning of the first group psychiatric practice. The Menninger School of Psychiatry, established shortly afterward in 1946, quickly became the country's largest training centre for psychiatric professionals, who were needed in increasing numbers to treat veterans returning home from World War II. About the same time, William Menninger led a national effort to reform state sanitariums; in 1948 he was featured on the cover of *Time* magazine, which hailed him as "psychiatry's U.S. sales manager."

Karl and William Menninger played guiding roles as the Menninger Foundation's activities and institutions grew and diversified. William served as medical director of the Menninger Psychiatric Hospital and as president of the Menninger Foundation. Karl founded and directed the Menninger School of Psychiatry from 1946 to 1969 and served as chairman of the board of trustees of the Menninger Foundation. He also published books that explored psychiatry's relation to society, and he wrote laypersons' guides to psychoanalytic theory. In 1974 the foundation established the Center for Applied Behavioral Sciences, which provided current scientific information on human behaviour and motivation to business, industry, and government.

Descendents of the two brothers continued their involvement with the Menninger Foundation and Clinic, although many of the clinic's operations were reduced in 2000. At a time when many institutions sought to reduce treatment costs, the psychoanalytical approach pioneered by the Menningers came to be seen as time consuming and expensive. In 2002 the Menninger Clinic coordinated its teaching and research activities with the Methodist Hospital and Baylor College of Medicine in Houston, Texas. In 2003 the clinic moved from Topeka to Houston, where it continued to provide a range of diagnostic and speciality inpatient programs for various age groups.

ANTONIA NOVELLO
(b. Aug. 23, 1944, Fajardo, Puerto Rico)

Physician and public official Antonia Novello (née Antonia Coello) was the first woman and the first Hispanic to serve as surgeon general of the United States (1990–93).

Antonia Coello suffered from a painful colon condition from birth until she underwent corrective surgery at age 18. This experience influenced her to train as a physician in order to help minimize suffering in others. After completing both her undergraduate work (1965) and her medical training (1970) at the University of Puerto Rico, she married Joseph R. Novello, then a navy flight surgeon and later a psychiatrist, author, and medical journalist. The couple moved to Ann Arbor, Michigan, where she did her internship and residency in pediatrics, followed by a fellowship in pediatric nephrology, at the University of Michigan Medical Center. She then completed a fellowship at Georgetown University Hospital in 1974–75 (and later joined the teaching staff) and earned a master's degree in public health from Johns Hopkins University in 1982.

Novello joined the staff of the National Institutes of Health in 1978, rising to the deputy directorship of the National Institute of Child Health and Human Development in 1986. In 1982 and 1983 she also served as a congressional fellow on the staff of the Labor and Human Resources Committee, advising the legislators on bills dealing with such health issues as organ transplants and cigarette warning labels. In 1990 President George Bush appointed her surgeon general of the United States. As head of the Public Health Service, she promoted an antismoking campaign and improved AIDS education and worked for better health care for minorities, women, and children. She left the post of surgeon general in 1993 and became a representative for the United Nations Children's Fund (UNICEF), where she continued to address women's and children's health issues, working to eliminate nutritional problems such as iodine deficiency and to prevent substance abuse and smoking.

In 1996 Novello was a visiting professor of health policy and management and the special director for community health policy at the Johns Hopkins University School of Hygiene and Public Health, where she guided the development of education and research programs designed to better the health of communities lacking adequate health care resources. In 1999 she became commissioner of the New York State Department of Health, the largest public health agency in the country. Following her appointment, she focused the department's efforts on improving programs such as Child Health Plus and Medicaid and on ensuring affordable health care for the people of New York. She served as state commissioner of health until 2007. Novello received numerous awards throughout her career, including the James Smithson Bicentennial Medal (2002).

SIR WILLIAM OSLER

(b. July 12, 1849, Bond Head, Canada West [now Ontario], Can.—d. Dec. 29, 1919, Oxford, Eng.)

Canadian physician and professor of medicine Sir William Osler practiced and taught in Canada, the United States, and Great Britain and was known for his work *The Principles and Practice of Medicine* (1892), which was a leading textbook. Osler played a key role in transforming the organization and curriculum of medical education, emphasizing the

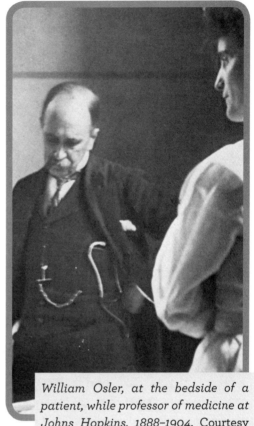

William Osler, at the bedside of a patient, while professor of medicine at Johns Hopkins, 1888–1904. Courtesy of the Osler Library, McGill University, Montreal

importance of clinical experience. He was created a baronet in 1911.

William Osler was the youngest of the nine children of the Reverend Featherstone Osler, who had gone to Canada as an Anglican missionary, and his wife, Ellen. William, like his father, was intended for the church. But while at school he became fascinated by natural history. He began to study at Trinity College, Toronto, but decided that the church was not for him and entered the Toronto Medical School in 1868. He subsequently transferred to McGill University in Montreal, Que., where he took his medical degree in 1872. During the following two years he visited medical centres in Europe, spending the longest period at University College, London, in the physiology laboratory of John Burdon-Sanderson, who was making experimental physiology preeminent in medical education.

In 1873 Osler demonstrated that hitherto unidentified bodies in the blood were in fact the third kind of blood corpuscles, which were later named the blood platelets. These corpuscles had been observed before, but no one before Osler had studied them so thoroughly. Thus began what he called his periods of "brain dusting"— travel and studies that made him almost as much a part of Europe as of America.

Osler returned to Canada and began general practice in Dundas but was soon appointed lecturer in the institutes of medicine at McGill University. He became professor there in 1875. A year later he became pathologist to the Montreal General Hospital and in 1878 physician to that hospital. At McGill he taught physiology, pathology, and medicine. His research was conducted largely in the postmortem room. In 1884 he was invited to occupy the chair of clinical medicine at the University of Pennsylvania in Philadelphia. He decided to do so on the toss of a coin. While in Philadelphia he became a founding member of the Association of American Physicians.

In 1888 Osler became the first professor of medicine in the new Johns Hopkins University Medical School in Baltimore. There he joined William H. Welch, chief of pathology, Howard A. Kelly, chief of gynecology and obstetrics, and William S. Halsted, chief of surgery. Together, the four transformed the organization and curriculum of clinical teaching and made Johns Hopkins the most famous medical school in the world. Students studied their patients in the wards and presented the results to the "Chief." They were also encouraged to take their problems to the laboratory. Finally, the experts pooled their knowledge for the benefit of the patient and the student in public teaching sessions. Thus was born the pattern of clinical teaching that spread throughout the United States. Osler was not only professor of medicine but physician in chief to the hospital, an office first devised by the president of the university on the basis of his experience of running a large department store and later to spread to most of the medical centres of the United States. For the first four years there were no students at Johns Hopkins, and Osler used the time to write *The Principles and Practice of Medicine,* first published in 1892. In the same year, he married Grace Gross, widow of a surgical colleague at Philadelphia and great-granddaughter of Paul Revere.

Osler's textbook was lucid, comprehensive, interesting, and scholarly. It quickly became the most popular medical textbook of its day and has continued to be published since under a succession of editors, though never regaining the quality with which Osler endowed it. The textbook had an unexpected sequel. In 1897 it was read by F.T. Gates, who had been engaged by John D. Rockefeller to advise him in his philanthropic endeavours. As a result of his reading, Gates inspired Rockefeller to direct his foundation toward medical research and to establish the Rockefeller Institute of Medical Research in New York.

In 1904, while visiting in England, Osler was invited to succeed Sir John Burdon-Sanderson in the Regius chair of medicine at the University of Oxford. Osler's practice and teaching had for many years imposed enormous demands on his time and energy. His forceful wife telegraphed him from America: "Do not procrastinate. Accept at once." Osler did. The Regius chair at Oxford is a crown appointment for which only citizens of the crown are eligible, but Osler had kept his Canadian nationality. He took up his chair in the autumn of 1905. In Oxford he taught only once a week, did a small amount of practice, and spent most of his time on his books. His library became one of the best of its kind, and after his death it passed intact to McGill, where it is specially housed. His scholarship was recognized by his election as president of the Classical Association. He was also active in medical affairs and inspired the formation of the Association of Physicians of Great Britain and Ireland and the establishment of the *Quarterly Journal of Medicine*. He was elected a fellow of the Royal College of Physicians of London in 1884 and a fellow of the Royal Society of London in 1898. He and his wife

were immensely hospitable, especially to visiting Americans, among whom their house was known as the "Open Arms."

Osler gave many lectures on medicine, some of which were collected and published. *Aequanimitas*, which he regarded as the most desirable quality for doctors, was the title of the most famous of these. Osler had a puckish wit and wrote some admirable medical nonsense under the pseudonym of Egerton Yorrick Davis, whom he presented as a retired surgeon captain of the U.S. Army.

In medical terminology, Osler is immortalized in Osler's nodes (red, tender swellings of the hand characteristic of certain cardiac infections), a blood disorder known as Osler-Vaquez disease, and Osler-Rendu-Weber disease (a hereditary disorder marked by recurring nose bleeds with vascular involvement of the skin and mucous membranes). The Oslers had one son, Revere, named after his great-great-grandfather, Paul Revere. His death in action during World War I took the spirit out of his father, who died of pneumonia in 1919.

MARY JANE SAFFORD
(b. Dec. 31, 1834, Hyde Park, Vt., U.S.—d. Dec. 8, 1891, Tarpon Springs, Fla.)

American physician Mary Jane Safford was known for her extensive nursing experience during the Civil War, which determined her on a medical career.

Safford grew up from the age of three in Crete, Illinois. During the 1850s she taught school while living with an older brother successively in Joliet, Shawneetown, and Cairo, Illinois. At the outbreak of the Civil War in the spring of 1861, Cairo became a town of some strategic importance because of its situation at the confluence of the Ohio and Mississippi rivers. The town was quickly occupied by volunteer troops from Chicago, and almost as quickly a variety of epidemic diseases broke out in the hastily constructed camps behind the levee. Safford began visiting the camps to tend the sick and to distribute food she had prepared. She gradually won the respect of officers and surgeons who had initially opposed her, and she was soon permitted to draw upon supplies collected and forwarded by the U.S. Sanitary Commission. By summer she was working closely with "Mother" Mary Ann Bickerdyke, who gave her some training in nursing. In November 1861 Safford nursed the wounded on the battlefield at Belmont, Missouri. In February 1862 she and Bickerdyke helped transport wounded from Fort Donelson to Cairo, and in April that year, following the Battle of Shiloh (Pittsburg Landing) in southwestern Tennessee, she worked aboard the hospital ship *Hazel Dell*. By that time her almost ceaseless labours had left her utterly exhausted, and she saw no more service during the war.

After an extended convalescent tour of Europe, Safford returned to the United States determined to become a physician. She graduated from the New York Medical College for Women in 1869 and then pursued advanced training in Europe for three years. At the University of Breslau, Germany (now Wrocław, Poland), she became the first woman to perform an ovariotomy. In 1872 she opened a private practice in Chicago. The next year, after her marriage to a Bostonian, she moved her practice to that city and became professor of women's diseases at the Boston University School of Medicine and a staff physician at the Massachusetts Homeopathic Hospital. She retired from medical practice in 1886.

DAVID SATCHER
(b. March 2, 1941, near Anniston, Ala.)

American medical doctor and public health administrator David Satcher was (1998–2002) the 16th surgeon general of the United States.

The son of a small farmer, Satcher nearly died of whooping cough at age two because his family had little access to health care. He was attended by the only black physician in the area and resolved from an early age to become a doctor. At his racially segregated high school, he was class valedictorian and was one of only three graduates to go on to college, earning a B.S. in 1963 from Morehouse College, a historically black institution in Atlanta, Georgia. In 1970 he became the first African American to earn both an M.D. and a Ph.D. (cytogenetics) at Case Western Reserve University in Cleveland, Ohio.

During the 1970s Satcher held administrative and teaching posts in Los Angeles at the Charles R. Drew Postgraduate Medical School and its

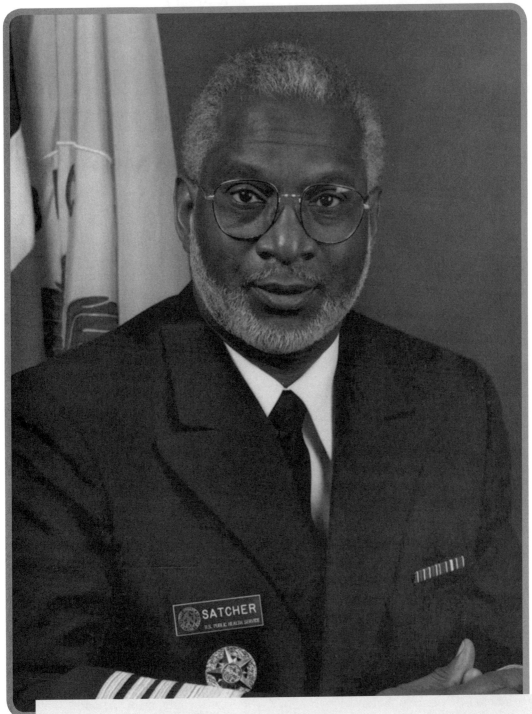

David Satcher. National Institutes of Health

affiliated hospital, the King-Drew Sickle Cell Center, and UCLA's School of Public Health. He returned to Morehouse in 1979 to chair the department of community medicine and family practice, and from 1982 to 1993 he served as president of Meharry Medical College in Nashville, Tennessee. When Satcher assumed the presidency, Meharry, dedicated to training African American doctors for 100 years, was on the verge of losing its accreditation; he recruited new faculty members, strengthened its academic standing, and ensured the financial security of both the school and its teaching hospital.

In 1993 Satcher was appointed director of the Centers for Disease Control and Prevention (CDC). During his tenure he emphasized disease prevention, instituting initiatives to raise childhood immunization rates, address emerging infectious diseases, and prevent food-borne illnesses. Satcher was appointed surgeon general by President Bill Clinton and assumed his duties in February 1998. Until January 2001 he served concurrently as assistant secretary of health in the Department of Health and Human Services. Together these positions provided a forum to emphasize public health issues and shape biomedical research policy. In his role as the nation's chief doctor, Satcher presented a report to the president on tobacco use (focusing on the health risks of smoking for minorities and minority teenagers), commissioned a report on suicide prevention, sought to eliminate race-based health care disparities,

and urged the nation to open an "honest debate" on mental health. In 2001 Satcher released a groundbreaking and controversial report titled *The Call to Action to Promote Sexual Health and Responsible Sexual Behavior*, which emphasized the role of research-based strategies in addressing issues related to sexual health.

After his term as surgeon general ended in February 2002, Satcher became director of the National Center for Primary Care at the Morehouse School of Medicine. He later served as president of the medical school from 2004 to 2006. His interest in improving public health policy and in cultivating leadership and diversity in the public health sector inspired him to develop the Satcher Health Leadership Institute at Morehouse School of Medicine in 2006. Satcher received many awards throughout his career, including the New York Academy of Medicine Lifetime Achievement Award (1997) and the Jimmy and Rosalynn Carter Award for Humanitarian Contributions to the Health of Humankind (1999).

MARIE STOPES

(b. Oct. 15, 1880, Edinburgh, Scot.—d. Oct. 2, 1958, near Dorking, Surrey, Eng.)

British advocate of birth control Marie Stopes founded the United Kingdom's first instructional clinic for contraception in 1921. Although her clinical work, writings, and speeches evoked violent opposition, especially from Roman Catholics, she greatly influenced the Church of

England's gradual relaxation (from 1930) of its stand against birth control.

Stopes grew up in a wealthy, educated family; her father was an architect, her mother a scholar of Shakespeare and an advocate for the education of women. Stopes obtained a science degree (1902) from University College, London, which she completed in only two years. She went on to do postgraduate studies in paleobotany (fossil plants), earning a doctorate from the University of Munich in 1904. That same year she became an assistant lecturer of botany at the University of Manchester. She specialized in fossil plants and the problems of coal mining. She married her first husband, a botanist named Reginald Ruggles Gates, in 1911. Stopes would later assert that her marriage was unconsummated and that she knew little about sex when she first married. Her failed marriage and its eventual annulment in 1916 played a large role in determining her future career, causing her to turn her attention to the issues of sex, marriage, and childbirth and their meaning in society. She initially saw birth control as an aid to marriage fulfillment and as a means to save women from the physical strain of excessive childbearing. In this regard for quality of life of the individual woman, she differed from most other early leaders of the birth-control movement, who were more concerned with social good, such as the elimination of overpopulation and poverty.

In 1918 Stopes married Humphrey Verdon Roe, cofounder of the A.V. Roe aircraft firm, who also had strong interests in the birth-control movement. He helped her in the crusade that she then began. Their original birth-control clinic—designed to educate women about the few methods of birth control available to them—was founded three years later, in the working-class Holloway district of London. That same year she became founder and president of the Society for Constructive Birth Control, a platform from which she spoke widely about the benefits of married women having healthy, desired babies. In the meantime she wrote *Married Love* and *Wise Parenthood* (both 1918), which were widely translated. Her *Contraception: Its Theory, History and Practice* (1923) was, when it first appeared, the most comprehensive treatment of the subject. After World War II she promoted birth control in East Asian countries.

HELEN BROOKE TAUSSIG
(b. May 24, 1898, Cambridge, Mass., U.S.—d. May 20, 1986, Kennett Square, Pa.)

American physician Helen Brooke Taussig was recognized as the founder of pediatric cardiology and is best known for her contributions to the development of the first successful treatment of "blue baby" syndrome.

Helen Taussig was born into a distinguished family as the daughter of Frank and Edith Guild Taussig. Her father was a prominent economics professor at Harvard University, and her mother was one of the first women to attend Radcliffe College (today known as the Radcliffe Institute for Advanced Study), an extension of Harvard that provided instruction for women. Although Taussig enjoyed a privileged upbringing, adversity cultivated in her a determination that later defined her character. As a child, the dyslexic Taussig laboured to become proficient in reading and was tutored by her father, who recognized the potential of her logical mind. When Taussig was 11, her mother died of tuberculosis, an illness Helen would later contract as well. However, these obstacles did not discourage Taussig from obtaining a university education. She enrolled at Radcliffe College in 1917, transferring to the University of California, Berkeley, in 1919, where she earned an A.B. in 1921. Taussig aspired to study medicine at Harvard but was denied admission because the university did not accept women into its academic degree program. Instead, she attended the Boston University School of Medicine from 1922 to 1924 and graduated from the Johns Hopkins University School of Medicine in 1927.

Two individuals had a far-reaching impact on Taussig's career. First was Canadian pathologist Maude Abbott of McGill University in Montreal. Abbott was a strong-minded role model whose earlier studies of congenital heart disease created the foundation for Taussig's own research into heart disease. Then, while an intern at Johns Hopkins, Taussig's work attracted the attention of American pediatrician Edwards A. Park, the director and, later, the chief of pediatrics at Johns Hopkins. In 1930 Park elevated Taussig to director of Hopkins' Harriet Lane Clinic, a health care centre for children, making her one of the first women in the country to hold such a prestigious position.

Taussig's career advanced, but her personal challenges mounted. In her 30s she grew deaf, and as a result she developed an innovative method to explore the beat of the human heart using her hands to compensate for her hearing loss. Relying on this method, Taussig noticed common beat patterns in the malformed hearts of infant patients who outwardly displayed a cyanotic hue and hence were known as "blue babies." She traced the root of the problem to a lack of oxygenated blood circulating from the lungs to the heart. Taussig reasoned that the creation of an arterial patent ductus, or shunt, would alleviate the problem, and she championed the cause before American surgeon Alfred Blalock, Hopkins' chief of the department of surgery. Together they developed the Blalock-Taussig shunt, an artery-like tube designed to deliver oxygen-rich blood from the lungs to the heart. On Nov. 29, 1944, Eileen Saxton, an infant affected by tetralogy of Fallot, a congenital heart disorder that gives rise to blue baby syndrome and that was previously considered untreatable, became the first patient to survive a successfully implanted Blalock-Taussig shunt. The miracle surgery was touted in the American magazines *Time* and *Life*, as well as in newspapers around the world. Later, American laboratory technician Vivien Thomas was also recognized for his contributions to the surgery.

Taussig was a prolific writer, publishing an astounding number of medical papers. In 1947 she wrote *Congenital Malformations of the Heart*, which was revised in 1960. Throughout her lifetime she received worldwide honours. She was awarded the Medal of Freedom by U.S. President Lyndon B. Johnson in 1964, and in 1965 Taussig became the first woman president of the American Heart Association. In addition, Taussig testified before the U.S. Congress about the harmful effects of the drug thalidomide, which had produced deformed children in Europe.

Taussig's ideas and determination have had long-lasting impacts on cardiology. Physicians originally believed the early blue babies could possibly endure a 40-year life span. At the turn of the 21st century, some of these early patients continued to survive into their sixth decade.

CONCLUSION

The growth of medicine from a practice based on supernatural phenomena to a field grounded in science was a gradual transition, taking centuries to be realized. The translation of ancient Greek medical texts by Arab scholars in the Middle Ages led to the subsequent adoption of Greek philosophy and scientific thought by the European scholars of the Renaissance and Enlightenment eras. It was this string of events that gave rise

to Western medicine and supported the later scientific research into all the various elements of health and disease—from the anatomical studies of Andreas Vesalius and the discovery of circulation by William Harvey to the verification of germ theory, the introduction of antibiotics, and breakthroughs in cancer research.

Along the way, there have been countless physicians and researchers contributing to the ever-expanding field of medicine. Some of these individuals developed new hypotheses and theories that broadened medical thinking. Others designed new instruments and methods for the diagnosis and treatment of disease. Still others were instrumental in effecting new health policies and in establishing medical institutions. It is the collective work of these individuals that has made Western medicine the entity known to so many people worldwide today.

Yet, despite the centuries of progress, it is widely acknowledged that modern medicine is not absolute. Indeed, the continued pursuit of unanswered questions in medical research and the improvement of existing technologies by future generations of scientists, physicians, and nurses remains indispensable to medicine. And in the singular endeavour of advancing the art of healing, the physicians of tomorrow tread common ground with their predecessors of centuries past.

GLOSSARY

acupuncture A form of traditional Chinese medicine involving the placement of fine needles at certain special points in the body. It is said to relieve a long list of health problems.

adrenaline A hormone that is secreted by the adrenal glands. Adrenaline, also known as epinephrine, is released during stressful or dangerous moments to help animals (including humans) focus and give them energy.

attenuated Weakened, or reduced in severity.

bacteria A single cell prokaryotic organism.

bile A yellow-greenish substance made in the liver that helps break down fat during the process of digestion.

chyle A milky mix of lymphatic fluid and fat released from food during the digestion process.

diphtheria A highly contagious bacterial disease that causes a thick membrane to form, often in the throat, and also spreads toxins around the body. It can cause inflammation of the heart and damage to the nervous system, as well as death.

deoxyribonucleic acid (DNA) A nucleic acid that contains the genetic instructions used in the development and functioning of all known living organisms and some viruses.

enteric Of or about the intestinal system.

epidemic An outbreak of disease that is highly prevalent in a fairly short period.

epilepsy Chronic neurological disorder characterized by sudden and recurrent seizures that are caused by excessive signaling of nerve cells in the brain.

etiology Related to how diseases are caused.

hemoglobin Iron-containing protein found in the red blood cells that transports oxygen to the tissues.

histology A branch of biology studying the organization and makeup of animal and plant tissues.

homeostasis A state of equilibrium or balance in body metabolism.

hormone A substance in both animals and plants that helps to regulate physical activities in the body and keep them stable.

humour In ancient and medieval physiology, four body fluids (blood, phlegm, black bile, and yellow bile) that determined people's temperaments and health by their relative proportions.

hypothyroidism A condition caused by a lack of adequate hormone production from the thyroid. It is characterized by slowness, sleepiness, weakness, and dry skin. In young children, it can cause intellectual disabilities or dwarfism.

materia medica A body of knowledge on medicines and their effects.

pandemic An epidemic that takes place over a widely spread area.

pathogenic Causing or capable of causing disease.

pathology A branch of medical studies related to discovering causes of disease and the effects of disease on living things.

philosopher's stone A legendary substance that alchemists believed could transform lead into gold or other precious metals.

phlegm Thick mucus in abnormal amounts.

plasma The fluid part of the blood, as differentiated from the suspended material (i.e., red blood cells, white blood cells, platelets, etc.).

protozoan Any member of the subkingdom Protozoa, a collection of single-celled eukaryotic organisms.

teleology An explanation that refers to some purpose or end.

virulent Something, such as a virus or bacteria, that can overwhelm a body's defense against disease.

BIBLIOGRAPHY

The literature on the history of medicine covers all topics and periods and includes biographies as well as descriptions of the development of hospitals, research institutes, health care, and medical education in different countries. Historical studies include George T. Bettany, *Eminent Doctors: Their Lives and Their Work*, 2 vol. (1885, reprinted 1972); Arturo Castiglioni, *A History of Medicine*, 2nd rev. ed. (1947; originally published in Italian, 1927), a classic work; Fielding H. Garrison, *An Introduction to the History of Medicine*, 4th rev. ed. (1929, reprinted 1967), a scholarly history; Douglas Guthrie, *A History of Medicine*, rev. ed. (1958); Howard W. Haggard, *Devils, Drugs, and Doctors: The Story of the Science of Healing from Medicine-Man to Doctor* (1929, reprinted 1980); Richard H. Meade, *An Introduction to the History of General Surgery* (1968), a well-documented work on developments in surgery on separate organs.

Modern overviews of the history of medicine and its practitioners include F. González-Crussi, *A Short History of Medicine*, vol. 28 of the Modern Library chronicles (2007); Philip Rhodes, *An Outline History of Medicine* (1985); and *The Oxford Companion to Medicine*, 3rd ed., edited by Stephen Lock, John M. Last, and George Dunea (2005).

Ancient traditions of medicine are presented in Steven B. Kayne, *Traditional Medicine: A Global Perspective* (2010); and Donald E. Kendall, *Dao of Chinese Medicine: Understanding an Ancient Healing Art* (2002).

For developments from the origin of Western medicine to the end of the 18th century, see William G. Black, *Folk-Medicine: A Chapter in the History of Culture* (1883, reprinted 1970); W.H.R. Rivers, *Medicine, Magic, and Religion* (1924, reprinted 1979), a comprehensive treatment of primitive medicine; Robert S. Gottfried, *Doctors and Medicine in Medieval England, 1340–1530* (1986); A. Wear, R.K. French, and I.M. Lonie (eds.), *The Medical Renaissance of the Sixteenth Century* (1985); Katharine Park, *Doctors and Medicine in Early Renaissance Florence* (1985); and Guy Williams, *The Age of Agony: The Art of Healing, c. 1700–1800* (1975, reprinted 1986).

The history of surgery is the subject of Harold Ellis, *The Cambridge Illustrated History of Surgery* (2009); and Knut Hæger, *The Illustrated History of Surgery* (2000).

Other works of interest, covering various aspects of the history of medicine, are Carl J. Pfeiffer, *The Art and Practice of Western Medicine in the Early Nineteenth Century* (1985); and Ruth J. Abram (ed.), *Send Us a Lady Physician: Women Doctors in America, 1835–1920* (1985).

INDEX